Studies in Computational Intelligence

Volume 685

Series editor

Janusz Kacprzyk, Polish Academy of Sciences, Warsaw, Poland
e-mail: kacprzyk@ibspan.waw.pl

About this Series

The series "Studies in Computational Intelligence" (SCI) publishes new developments and advances in the various areas of computational intelligence—quickly and with a high quality. The intent is to cover the theory, applications, and design methods of computational intelligence, as embedded in the fields of engineering, computer science, physics and life sciences, as well as the methodologies behind them. The series contains monographs, lecture notes and edited volumes in computational intelligence spanning the areas of neural networks, connectionist systems, genetic algorithms, evolutionary computation, artificial intelligence, cellular automata, self-organizing systems, soft computing, fuzzy systems, and hybrid intelligent systems. Of particular value to both the contributors and the readership are the short publication timeframe and the worldwide distribution, which enable both wide and rapid dissemination of research output.

More information about this series at http://www.springer.com/series/7092

Katarzyna A. Tarnowska
Zbigniew W. Ras · Pawel J. Jastreboff

Decision Support System for Diagnosis and Treatment of Hearing Disorders

The Case of Tinnitus

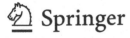 Springer

Katarzyna A. Tarnowska
Department of Computer Science
University of North Carolina at Charlotte
Charlotte, NC
USA

Pawel J. Jastreboff
Department of Otolaryngology
Emory University School of Medicine
Atlanta, GA
USA

Zbigniew W. Ras
Department of Computer Science
University of North Carolina at Charlotte
Charlotte, NC
USA

ISSN 1860-949X ISSN 1860-9503 (electronic)
Studies in Computational Intelligence
ISBN 978-3-319-84657-6 ISBN 978-3-319-51463-5 (eBook)
DOI 10.1007/978-3-319-51463-5

This Springer imprint is published by Springer Nature
The registered company is Springer International Publishing AG
The registered company address is: Gewerbestrasse 11, 6330 Cham, Switzerland

Preface

This book describes RECTIN (Recommender System for Tinnitus)—system supporting a physician in tinnitus patients' diagnosis and treatment. The work verifies a hypothesis about a possibility of building such a system for the specific needs of medical facility following treatment protocol of Tinnitus Retraining Therapy. It examines possibility of using information technology, in particular methods of data mining and machine learning, in the field of medicine and practical applications of recommendation systems in the field.

The book introduces the topic of tinnitus as a problem area, shows the basic concepts of Recommender Systems (RS), its current state of the art and their real-world applications in different areas, focusing on Health RS. It proposes knowledge discovery approach for decision support system development and presents theoretical concepts and algorithms for rule-based systems, including: decision tables, classification rules, action rules extraction and meta actions. Empirical part includes: description of a raw dataset of tinnitus patients and visits, provided by Dr. P. Jastreboff from Emory University School of Medicine in Atlanta, applied data preprocessing techniques and results from experiments on classification and action rules extraction from the cleansed dataset.

Charlotte, USA
May 2016

Katarzyna A. Tarnowska
Zbigniew W. Ras
Pawel J. Jastreboff

Contents

Chapter 1
Introduction

Abstract Recently, there has been an increasing interest in business analytics and big data tools to understand and drive industries evolution. The healthcare industry is also interested in new methods to analyze data and provide better care. Given the wealth of data that various institutions are accumulating, it is natural to take advantage of data driven decision-making solutions. Recommender systems proved to be a valuable mean to deal with the decision problems, especially in commercial merchandising. They are of special importance nowadays, when people are facing information overload and the growth and variety of information (products, news) available on the Web frequently overwhelms individuals. It leads them, in turn, to make poor decisions and decreases their well-being. Recommender systems enable automation of some of strategies in human decision making, support their users in various processes, providing advice that is both high-quality and high-personalized. In the area of healthcare they provide valuable support for physicians treating their patients, such as the one described in [Szl15]. The potential economic benefits of applying computerized clinical decision support systems include improved efficiency in health care delivery e.g. by reducing costs as well as improved quality of care and improved patient safety.

1.1 Objective

The goal of this research work is to design and describe Recommender System for Diagnosis and Treatment of Tinnitus (in short Recommender for Tinnitus, or RECTIN)—a system supporting a doctor in a decision making process, with regard to categorization of a patient and in choice of particular methods of treatment.

The main motivation for taking up the topic is to study and analyze the possibilities of applying modern information technologies and machine learning methods in the area of medicine and practical use of recommender systems in such settings. This

© Springer International Publishing AG 2017
K.A. Tarnowska et al., *Decision Support System for Diagnosis and Treatment of Hearing Disorders*, Studies in Computational Intelligence 685,
DOI 10.1007/978-3-319-51463-5_1

work should verify the hypothesis that such system can be built within the chosen methodology and successfully used for the needs of doctors dealing with tinnitus. It should ultimately contribute to the better effectiveness and efficiency of tinnitus treatment.

The design of a model of artificial advisor will be based on building a prototype of a recommender system with the use of the chosen technologies. The system should give diagnostic recommendations, driven by classification rules, and treatment recommendations, driven by action rules. The rules for the knowledge base of the recommender system will be extracted with the use of data mining/machine learning methods applied on the dataset of tinnitus patients and visits. The dataset is provided by doctor Jastreboff from Emory University School of Medicine in Atlanta, who specializes in tinnitus and developed a successful method for its treatment called Tinnitus Retraining Therapy.

Machine learning and data exploration methods should help in understanding relationships among the treatment factors and audiological measurements along with changing patient emotions, in order to better understand tinnitus treatment. Additionally, different preprocessing techniques will be used, including text mining and clustering, so that to transform the tinnitus dataset into more suitable for machine understanding.

1.2 Organization of this Book

This chapter (this introduction) presents main goals, motivation and the research scope of this book.

Chapter 2 is an introduction to the problem area, which will be solved and supported with the recommender system—tinnitus treatment and characterization. In the face of challenges associated with human problem solving, it postulates the need for building such system in the given application area. It describes a process (a protocol of the TRT treatment), which should be modeled by a computer program.

Chapter 3 is a general overview and state of the art of recommender systems technology, developed in recent years, applied in different areas, along with examples in the commercial settings. It describes different approaches to build RS, discusses benefits and disadvantages of each of them, and finally helps in motivating the choice of an approach suitable for the problem being solved within this work.

Chapter 4 presents theoretical background for building a knowledge-based recommender system in a greater detail, discussing methods of extracting and applying rules for solving a problem of tinnitus treatment. It focuses on concepts and algorithms for action rules and meta actions. The knowledge discovery approach is presented in the context of its potential to build a knowledge engine for RS (as decision rules constitute the diagnostic module and action rules—module for recommending treatment).

Chapter 5 provides an overview and design project of the RECTIN system (Recommender for Tinnitus)—the ultimate goal of the work within this project. It lists the main components of the systems and their functionalities. The functionalities are presented in relation to the supported processes in a medical facility, with the main use cases for the system. The chapter also describes a dataset of tinnitus patients and their visits, which serves as a knowledge base of the system. It introduces initial preprocessing steps performed on raw data, collected by authors. Next chapters present methodologies of developing each of the component in a greater detail.

Chapter 6 is an elaboration on classification module development and presents outcomes of the experiments on choosing the best prediction method for the cleansed dataset. It also presents first attempts with developing features that could be relevant to the tinnitus characterization. It concludes with comparison on experiments with different preprocessing and prediction methods, suggesting the final choice for implementation.

Chapter 7 is dedicated to description of experiments on association rule extraction. It presents selectively outcome rules as hypotheses, generated from the tinnitus dataset with the use of the chosen data mining tool. It assesses reliability of the rules along with their viability to be implemented into RECTIN knowledge base.

Chapter 8 focuses on action rule discovery. Further preprocessing techniques are described, as well as methods in dealing with missing data. It provides analysis (interpretation) of sample rules generated by data mining tasks.

Chapter 9 is an elaboration on the previous one, providing description on further enhancements on attribute development and designed algorithms on missing data imputation. It concludes with final choice of most reliable rules to be implemented within RECTIN rule engine. It also provides a summary of experiments on rules extraction with the chosen methodology.

Chapter 10 presents RECTIN prototype implementation of each system component: application, transactional database, classification module and rule engine. The last mentioned module is described along with algorithm on rule execution and method for rule declaration in the system.

Chapter 11 is a final conclusion of the work done within this project, discussing the possibilities of its further extension.

Chapter 2
Tinnitus Treatment as a Problem Area

Abstract This chapter presents the decision problem area which will be supported with a recommender system technology, that is, tinnitus diagnosis and treatment. It will introduce the problem of tinnitus and next, the successful method of treatment applied by doctor P. Jastreboff. At the end of this chapter major results from the treatment will be showed, along with possible new challenges, which can be handled with the help of information technology.

2.1 Tinnitus

2.1.1 Problem Description

Tinnitus, often described as "ringing in the ears", is a serious problem affecting a significant portion of population nowadays. According to our medical knowledge, it is important to differentiate between people who "experience" tinnitus from those who suffer because of it. According to some estimations, about 10–20% of general population is affected—in other words—they experience tinnitus—(in the USA it accounts to about 25–50 million people) and close to 90% had experienced from at least temporary tinnitus. It is most common in the group age of above 65 years old (tinnitus is reported by about 30% people in this age group). Certain occupational populations are high at risk of developing tinnitus: military personnel, police officers and firefighters, but also patients, who are undergoing ear-related surgery. Soldiers returning from Iraq or Afghanistan who where exposed to a blast noise, are reporting tinnitus in 49% of cases [MLDK10]. This also has financial implications: the American Veteran Administration spent $ 1.1 billion in 2009 on compensation for tinnitus alone, and it was expected to reach $2.3 billion by 2014 [MLDK10].

Only about 20% of those experiencing tinnitus, that is about 4–8% of general population suffer because of it—has prolonged tinnitus, moderately or significantly

© Springer International Publishing AG 2017

K.A. Tarnowska et al., *Decision Support System for Diagnosis and Treatment of Hearing Disorders*, Studies in Computational Intelligence 685, DOI 10.1007/978-3-319-51463-5_2

annoying, causing them to seek help (they are labeled as having clinically significant tinnitus) [JJ00]. In the UK, for example, currently, it affects around 10% of adults, and for about 1% it is so severe so that deteriorates a quality of their life (they have tinnitus with debilitating results [Web15]).

Causes of tinnitus are often not clear. It is associated with hearing loss, ear infections, acoustic neuroma, Menere's syndrome, and aging. It can be also a side-effect of some drugs. There is no cure for it and treatment methodologies prove ineffective in many cases, accompanied by significant side-effects or fail to provide systematic relief to patients. Also methods of treatment that work well for some patients, are not necessary effective for the others (therapies must be highly personalized).

2.1.2   Medical Background

The common understanding of tinnitus is a noise in the ears or head, described by the affected, as ringing, buzzing, humming, hissing, the sound of escaping steam, etc. [JJ00]. Tinnitus is more formally defined as "a phantom auditory perception, namely perception of sounds that results exclusively from activity within the nervous system without any corresponding mechanical, vibratory activity within cochlea, and not related to stimulation of any kind" [JH04]. This translates to a real perception of sound, for which there is no corresponding physical correlate. It can be compared to phantom limb and phantom pain phenomena. Tinnitus is often accompanied by decreased sound tolerance, consisting of hyperacusis,[1] misophonia.[2] Some patients exhibit phonophobia, which is a specific version of misophonia when fear is dominant factor.

Tinnitus-related neuronal activity (labeled in this chapter as tinnitus signal) is perceived as a sound. The tinnitus signal, perceived as a sound, is that of a neural activity somewhere in the brain. It is not exactly known, where in the brain this occurs, but some recent studies have indicated the secondary auditory cortex, as playing an important role in this. In 2015, for the first time, tinnitus signals have been mapped across the brain of a patient undergoing a surgery [Web15]. Previous experiments have been conducted with fMRI technique, which is nevertheless much less precise than recording electrical activity of the bran via electrodes inserted into the cortex. This method is, on the other hand, much more invasive, but in this case the electrodes were used for epilepsy monitoring, from which the patient happened to suffer, along with tinnitus, and on which he was operated.

As Fig. 2.1 shows, the tinnitus the patient is hearing correlates not only with a small area of auditory cortex, but throughout a huge proportion of the brain areas. It

---

[1] Commonly known as "discomfort to sounds", defined as an abnormally high level of sound induced activity occurring within auditory pathways, due to an abnormal amplification of sound-evoked neural signals [JJ06].

[2] The phenomenon of an overall negative attitude toward sound. Reflects an abnormally strong reaction of the limbic and autonomous system to sound without abnormally high activation of the auditory system [JJ06].

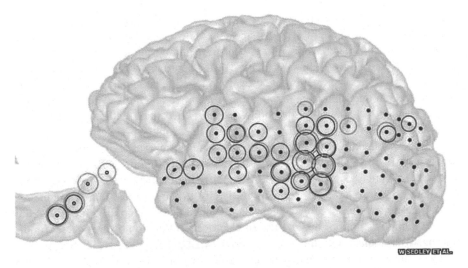

Fig. 2.1 The areas in the brain activity correlating with the heard tinnitus [Web15]

should, however, be taken into account that the data comes from one tinnitus patient only and the condition can vary.

2.2 Tinnitus Retraining Therapy

Tinnitus Retraining Therapy is a method proposed by Dr. Pawel Jatreboff, which is based on neurophysiological model of tinnitus [JJ00]. The method proved to have a very high success rate, although TRT does not cure tinnitus (tinnitus perception is still present). Method is based at retraining functional connections between the auditory system and other system in the brain, including limbic and autonomic nervous systems (but not only these two systems).

According to our medical experience [JJ00] this methodology is not only high-effective, but also does not have side-effects, requires limited amount of time and can be used on all of the patients disregarding etiology of tinnitus.

2.2.1 Neurophysiological Model

The definition of tinnitus proposed by Jastreboff stresses the involvement of a nervous system as a key component responsible for the emergence of tinnitus [JJ00]. Tinnitus is a result from not only neural activity in the auditory pathways, but as symptoms include anxiety, annoyance, strong emotional reactions, also involves activation of limbic and autonomic nervous systems as well as other systems in the brain. Thus the focus of the problem should be moved from the cochlea to the central nervous system. The first mentioned system—limbic—controls emotions and mood, for example, fear, thirst, hunger, joy and happiness, as well as motivation behaviors. Furthermore, it activates the second mentioned system-autonomic, which is responsible for basic organism functions, such as breathing, heart rate and hormones (action of glands). The Tinnitus Retraining Therapy is focused on the neurophysiology of these systems. Its main objective is habituation of activation of sympathetic part of the autonomic nervous system and therefore, habituation of negative reactions evoked by tinnitus and subsequently habituation of tinnitus perception occurs, without need for any specific treatment. It removes factors worsening the problem—negative feelings and emotions associated with it. On the other hand, most previous approaches and treatments were focused on removing, or at least decreasing tinnitus perception (tinnitus source), but were not very successful [MLDK10]. For example, one of such methods was based on introducing a medication directly to the cochlea. Other treatments, aiming at suppressing tinnitus perception, included using external sound that could "mask" tinnitus signal or making use of electrical stimulation of the cochlea, auditory nerve or recently even the auditory cortex [MLDK10]. All these methods proved either unsuccessful or only partially successful, low rate of success between 10 and 50%. Tinnitus treatments have high placebo effect which has been shown to be 40%.

Neurophysiology model, as depicted in the Fig. 2.2, was developed by Dr. Jastreboff in the 1980s. It stresses the auditory system as secondary only, and other systems in the brain, as dominant in clinically significant tinnitus [JJ00]. According to the model, the generation of tinnitus-related neuronal activity starts in the periphery of the auditory system (the cochlea, auditory nerve). The detection occurs in the subcortical auditory centers, and the perception (or interpretation)—at cortical areas. The confirmation for that is a study presented in [Web15] (see Fig. 2.1). It shows that different areas of brain are activated before the tinnitus signal reaches the level of conscious perception. The process of detection is accompanied by the sustained activation of the limbic (emotional) and autonomous nervous system. The last occurs only when a person concurrently experiences negative emotions (anxiety, psychoso-

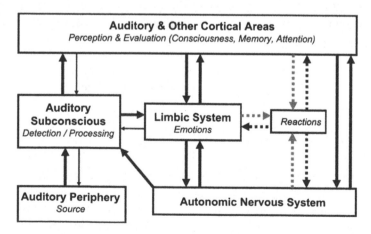

Fig. 2.2 The neurophysiological model of tinnitus [MLDK10]

matic reactions, annoyance) with their tinnitus. It is the factor causing distress and consequently, clinically relevant tinnitus. The patients with abnormally activation of limbic and autonomous systems experience stress, anxiety, loss of well-being leading them to greater annoyance with their tinnitus. Feedback loops connecting the auditory, limbic and autonomic nervous systems (see Fig. 2.2) are getting stronger, and patients continue to get worse [JJ00]. The creation and sustaining of connections between those systems are governed by the rules of conditioned reflexes (they link sensory stimulus with reaction) [JJ06]. The tinnitus signal in the auditory pathways acts as a conditioning stimulus, which via one or more reflex arc, activates the limbic and autonomous nervous systems and thus evokes negative reactions [MLDK10]. The increase in annoyance and anxiety also depends on patient's psychological profile, their association of tinnitus with something negative and not the psychoacoustic characteristic of the perceived sound of the tinnitus. In contrary, in case of hyperacusis, the reaction depends solely on the physical characteristics of a bothersome sound (such as its energy and frequency spectrum) [MLDK10]. In misophonia, on the other hand, adverse reactions occur due to specific patterns of sound. Most individuals with tinnitus experience just a sound sensation, but a part of them have negative reactions evoked by tinnitus. In the severe cases, patients may no longer enjoy any activities previously pleasant to them, which in turn may lead to depression. Patients who experienced "negative counseling" (that is statements such as "nothing can be done"; "you will have to learn to live with it"; "you have a bad brain") can further develop negative associations of their tinnitus, which triggers the development of a vicious cycle. "Negative counseling" is an example of reinforcement that creates conditioned reflex, which, in turns, creates physiological and behavioral reactions. Another common scenario of creating conditioned reflex is that, when a person experiences a strong emotionally negative stress situation, such as during retirement or divorce.

2.2.2 Habituation

According to Dr. Jastreboff, the presented neurophysiology model offers an approach to treat tinnitus [JJ00]. Though there is no cure for the source of tinnitus, the brain exhibits a high level of plasticity. Doctor claims that it is possible to induce habituation of tinnitus by interfering with tinnitus-related neuronal activity above its source. He proposes blocking the spread of the tinnitus signal to other than auditory regions of the brain, particularly to the limbic and autonomous nervous systems. It means that such successfully treated person will still perceive their tinnitus, but it will not bother them [MLDK10]. This is what is called 'habituation' of reactions, and is based on the principle that every conditioned reflex can be extinguished (retrained), when the reinforcement is not given (i.e., passive extinction of conditioned reflexes) or when positive reinforcement is associated with stimulus (i.e., active extinction of conditioned reflexes) and the reaction previously evoked by sensory stimulus can be abolished or modified [JJ06]. Habituation is a fundamental property of the brain function resulting from the fact, that the brain cannot handle more than one conscious task at a time (for example listening to two people talking at the same time). It

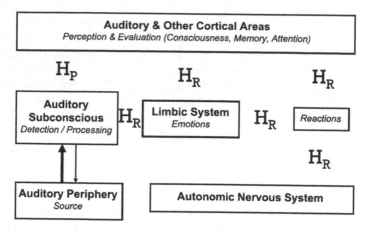

Fig. 2.3 The illustration of habituation of reactions (HR) and perception (HP) [MLDK10]

selects and blocks signals at a subconscious level on the basis of previous experience. Retraining/extinction of conditioned reflexes cannot be done on the cognitive level.

Habituation of tinnitus based on neurophysiologic model (Fig. 2.3) has two main goals: to habituate reactions of the limbic and autonomous nervous systems (to block tinnitus-related neural activity from reaching these systems) and to habituate perception (to block tinnitus-related neural activity before reaching the level of awareness). The first goal aims at relieving patients from negative reactions of their brain and the body associated with tinnitus. Counseling should be performed individually (tailored to individual needs), not as a group therapy. The final goal of the treatment, is that tinnitus ceases to have an impact on the patient's life.

Habituation is achieved by a variety of methods, including counseling and sound therapy. In order to be called Tinnitus Retraining Therapy, the treatment must involve both counseling and sound therapy (which involves providing the auditory system with enriched stimulation to decrease the contrast between tinnitus-related and background neuronal activity and consequently decreasing the strength of tinnitus signal). The classical approach for an extinction of conditional reflex would be to expose the subject to the same signal (tinnitus), while removing reinforcement. As tinnitus-related signals cannot be manipulated directly, another method is to decrease both the tinnitus signal (by sound therapy) and reinforcement (by reclassifying tinnitus to neutral stimuli—counseling) at the same time.

2.3 Treatment Protocol

The treatment protocol within TRT is composed of several steps:

- the initial appointment,
- audiological evaluation,
- medical evaluation,

- diagnosis with decision as for treatment,
- counseling.

The initial contact with a patient is made through a form (see Appendix A), which is then further expanded by an interview. The interview helps in identifying resulting problems, determining the impact of tinnitus on the patient's life and assessing the level of emotional distress. The audiological evaluation is performed starting with an otoscopic examination of the ear canal and tympanic membrane and a series of hearing tests, from which the most important outcomes are audiogram and LDL (loudness discomfort level). The medical evaluation of the patients aims, in the first place, at excluding any known medical condition that has tinnitus as one of its symptoms (the most common such conditions are: acoustic neuroma, Meniere's disease and otosclerosis).

2.3.1   Patient Categories

After the evaluation, a patient is placed into one of five categories, based on four factors (Table 2.1):

- the extent of impact tinnitus has on one's life (reflecting the strength of functional connections between the auditory system and the limbic and autonomous nervous systems),
- patient's subjective perception of hearing loss,
- presence or absence of hyperacusis (increased sensitivity to sounds),
- prolonged worsening of hyperacusis and/or tinnitus following exposure to moderate or loud sounds.

Category 0

Denotes patients with neither hyperacusis nor significant hearing loss, and whose tinnitus has little impact on their lives. In these cases, counseling sessions are sufficient and there is no need for any instrumentation.

Category 1

Patients (the most common category) have significant tinnitus, but without hyperacusis and hearing loss. They are treated, besides full counseling, with the use of sound generators set at the level close to "mixing" or "blending" point.[3]

---

[3]The level where partial suppression ("partial masking") starts to occur [MLDK10].

Table 2.1 Determining categories of tinnitus patients [JJ00]

Category	Hyperacusis	Prolonged sound-induced exacerbation	Subjective hearing loss	Impact on life	Treatment
0	–	–	–	Low	Counseling only
1	–	–	–	High	Sound generator set at mixing point
2	–	–	Present	High	Hearing aid with stress on enrichment of the auditory background
3	Present	–	Not relevant	High	Sound generators set above threshold of hearing
4	Present	Present	Not relevant	High	Sound generators set at threshold; very slow increase of sound level

Category 2

Consists of patients with the characteristics of *Category 1*, but additionally significant subjective hearing loss. These are advised to wear hearing aids, while enriching their sound environment. Currently, due to changes in hearing aids industry, the combination instruments (hearing aid and sound generators in one shell) become widely available and are predominant devices used for this category of patients.

Category 3

This category is used for patients with a significant hyperacusis that is not enhanced for a prolonged period of time. Sound generators are recommended for treating these patients. The sound level should be set below a level which would induce discomfort.

Category 4

This category denotes patients who have tinnitus and hyperacusis that is getting worse, when exposed to the sound. This category is the most difficult to treat. In this case, the sound generators, used in the treatment, are set to the threshold of hearing. As the treatment progresses, the sound level is increased slowly.

2.4   Motivation for RS Project

In summary, the TRT proves to be a very effective method, for both tinnitus and hyperacusis, and provides many other benefits [JJ00]:

- can be used to treat all patients,
- does not require frequent visits,
- does not interfere with hearing,
- there are no negative side-effects.

For majority of patients treated with this method, tinnitus constituted no longer a problem in their lives.

2.4.1   Treatment Results

TRT works independent of the cause of the tinnitus and can be successfully used for any type of tinnitus. The neurophysiological model of tinnitus has been proved in practice by results of clinical studies [MLDK10]. Many studies have been published on the effect of TRT, including systematic clinical trials and showed improvement in over 80% of the patients, and what is more, the improvement has proved to be persistent.

The treatment requires a significant amount of time (from 9 to 24 months) to provide steady development of plastic changes in the nervous system (habituation of tinnitus). It still does not guarantee 100% success rate. For the treatment to be effective it is necessary to retrain the feedback loops formed between the auditory, limbic and autonomous systems during consecutive follow-up visits. As a result, habituation decreases the strength of those connections. Patients are asked to asses their tinnitus awareness, annoyance and effect on life on a scale of 0–10 before and after treatment, as well as after each visit. The changes can be observed by comparing the initial form with the follow-up forms (see Appendices A and B). According to our medical expertise, the process of habituation is slow and characterized by fluctuations. Patients experience temporary tinnitus relief (due to partial habituation), but when it returns to its previous state, they perceive it as worsening. Initial improvement can be seen within few months, then follows the constant, gradual improvement. Clearer results can be seen on average after 3 months of therapy, but the doctor recommends that the treatment lasts at least 9 months. Doctor Jastreboff reported the effects of treatment on sample of 263 patients [JJ00]. About 90% of them received instruments (82.5% sound generators and 7.6% hearing aids). 9.9% received one session of counseling (and did not typically follow TRT). Results obtained from treatment on the patients revealed that 75% of them reported significant improvement. And the results (80%) were even more optimistic for patients who also were prescribed noise generators or hearing aids. On the average, the values for awareness, annoyance and life impact metrics decreased by half in comparison to their pre-treatment values. Also the patients from Categories 3 and 4 (that is those, who also suffered from hyperacusis) showed even greater improvement than patients with tinnitus only (categories 1 and 2). The method provided steady improvement after even after 3 or 5 years from ending the treatment [JJ06].

However, we must remember, that TRT is not a cure, but a treatment that allows patients to control their tinnitus and thus live a normal life and participate in everyday activities. TRT has been used clinically since 1988 and underwent many modifications since its first description. The method has not a stagnant protocol, but continues to evolve on the basis of information gathered from both treatment of patients and animal search findings [MLDK10].

2.4.2 Patient Dataset

The progress of treatment with Tinnitus Retraining Therapy (habituation of tinnitus) was monitored and collected in Tinnitus and Hyperacusis Center at Emory University School of Medicine. Original sample of 555 patients, described by forms during initial or follow-up visits, collected by Dr. Jastreboff, was used. Additionally, the Tinnitus Handicap Inventory (see Appendix C) was administered to individuals during their visits to the Center. The second database was extended to 758 patients [Tho11] (not made available), containing also a new form called *Tinnitus Functional Index*, or TFI, in shortcut. These databases, consisting of tuples identified with patient and visit numbers, have been developed over years by inserting patients' information from paper forms (developed by Dr. Jastreboff).

2.4.3 Problems with Human Approach

There remain some challenges in using the method with human approach. Evaluating results of tinnitus treatment is a challenge itself, because there exists no objective method for detecting the presence, the extent and severity of tinnitus, and there is also a high level of "placcbo effect" [JJ06]. Furthermore, the methodology has to be highly individualized to specific patient's profile and needs, sound generators must generate sounds that would not cause annoyance for a particular patient. Besides, it is often not clear, why particular technique proved to be successful in one case, while not in another case. The evaluation of any tinnitus treatment outcome is based on subjective evaluation of the problem. As a result of it, this treatment requires a lot of time and involvement from the personnel side, who has to be also specifically trained. Taking into account time restrictions in today's medical practice and the need for more efficient evaluation of different treatment methods, a proposal to develop a decision support tool besides forms, seems encouraging. It could also potentially provide more precision and objectivity, when dealing with tinnitus problem.

TRT is a complex treatment process, which generates a high volume of matrix data over time: some attributes have relatively stable values while others may be subject to change as the doctors are tuning the treatment parameters while symptoms of patients are altering [ZRJT10]. The medical dataset is sparse and has large volumes of missing variables for each patient. Many important clinical conditions are also poorly understood and associated with complex, multi-factorial conditions. Taking into account the requirement for making personalized recommendations and care to patients, the proposed computer-assisted treatment approach seems promising. Modern computing techniques, including machine learning, intelligent data analysis and recommender systems technologies, provide a new promising way to better understand, further improve and support the treatment. Understanding the relationships between patterns among treatment factors would help to optimize the treatment process.

Chapter 3
Recommender Solutions Overview

Abstract This chapter aims at providing an overview of RS technology, describing different types of RS, with emphasis on choosing the right approach for the system supporting tinnitus treatment and justifying particular choice. Current generation of recommendation methods is presented in division to four main categories:

- collaborative,
- content-based,
- knowledge-based,
- hybrid.

The chapter introduces basic concepts of each type, along with their mathematical/algorithmic foundations and general system architectures. The last section compares these different approaches with regard to requirements for tinnitus therapy recommendation and provides motivation to choose the rule-based approach for building a recommender system for the given problem area.

3.1 Recommender Systems Concept

Recommender systems are software tools and techniques that aim at suggesting hopefully useful items to users [KRRS11]. 'Item' is understood as anything that systems recommend to users, e.g., CDs, books or news, or, as in case of tinnitus—treatment method. In their simplest, personalized recommendations are presented as ranked list of items. This ranking is generated by applying prediction algorithms, based on the user's preferences and constraints. User preferences can be collected either explicitly, by interacting with user, or implicitly, by tracking the users' behavior.

Recommender Systems development involves expertise from different fields, such as: Artificial intelligence, Human Computer Interaction, Information Technology, Data Mining, Statistics, Adaptive User Interfaces, Decision Support Systems, Marketing, or Consumer Behavior [JZFF10]. In comparison to other classical

© Springer International Publishing AG 2017
K.A. Tarnowska et al., *Decision Support System for Diagnosis and Treatment of Hearing Disorders*, Studies in Computational Intelligence 685,
DOI 10.1007/978-3-319-51463-5_3

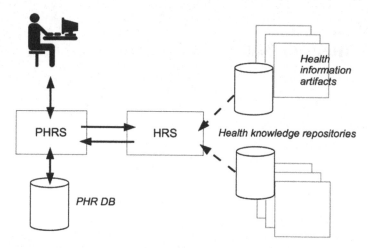

Fig. 3.1 Components of a PHR system with extension of an HRS [WP14]

information system tools and techniques, such as databases or search engines, the study of recommender systems is relatively new. It emerged as an independent research area in the mid-1990s, but interest in it increased dramatically over recent time. Now they are successfully deployed as a part of many e-commerce sites, offering several important business benefits: increasing the number of items sold, selling more diverse items, increasing user satisfaction and loyalty, helping to understand what the user wants.

3.1.1   Health Recommender Systems

Although being mostly developed in e-commerce, RS have been also recently adapted for medical purposes. The main goal is to assist physicians in making decisions without directly consulting specialists.

A *Health Recommender System* (HRS), as proposed in [WP14], is a specialized RS, where a recommendable item of interest is a piece of medical information, which itself is not linked to an individual's medical history. These suggestions are driven by individualized health data, such as, documented in a so-called *personal health record* (PHR), which can be considered a "user profile" of a recommender system. Such HRS is implemented as an extension of an existing PHR system, where data entries exist in a PHR database (DB) (as depicted in Fig. 3.1). When supplied with medical facts, an HRS computes a set of potentially relevant items of interest for a target user (for example an authorized health professional).

The paper [SK13] proposed to apply a Medical Recommender System for Telemedicine, thus, assisting community hospitals in remote areas of Thailand that have not only insufficient physicians, who usually have not enough abilities and

Evidence-based Medical Recommender Systems

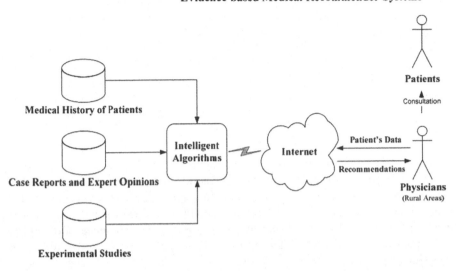

Fig. 3.2 Conceptual diagram of evidence-based medical recommender systems for telemedicine in Thailand [SK13]

experiences to diagnose all types of diseases, but also insufficient infrastructure. The architecture of the proposed system is presented in Fig. 3.2.

The system [SK13] implements intelligent algorithms, such as neural network, fuzzy theories, support vector machine, data mining techniques. It utilizes the hybrid filtering techniques: collaborative, content-based, and knowledge-based filtering. The collaborative filtering method is applied for medical history of patients; the content-based filtering is used for experimental studies, and the knowledge-based filtering is applied for the case reports and expert opinions. The physicians can access the system anywhere the Internet is available. The recommendations are delivered to the physicians based on their patients' physical examination, and then the physicians consult the patients for their diagnosis.

3.2 Collaborative Recommendation

The most common approach (used by many real online bookstores, for example) is to consider the behavior, opinions, and tastes of a large community of other users (or patients in HRS), for generating personalized recommendations. *Collaborative filtering* technique, used in this approach, leverages recommendations produced by a community of users to deliver recommendations to an *active user* (current patient). It is sometimes referred as 'people-to-people correlation'. It is based on the fact, that individuals often rely on recommendations provided by their peers in making daily decisions, and that similar people have similar tastes (or patients with similar characteristics and symptoms are approached with similar treatment). CF techniques require no domain knowledge and can be used on very sparse data [HS10].

Table 3.1 Example of input database for collaborative recommendation [JZFF10]

	Item1	Item2	Item3	Item4	Item5
Alice	5	3	4	4	?
User1	3	1	2	3	3
User2	4	3	4	3	5
User3	3	3	1	5	4
User4	1	5	5	2	1

The typical input for such systems is a matrix of given user-item ratings (see Table 3.1) and typical output is either a prediction indicating to what degree the current user will like or dislike a certain item (to which degree a treatment method is suitable for a patient) or a list of n recommended items. One of the earliest method used for this approach is called *user-based nearest neighbor recommendation*. First step in this method is identifying *peer users* or *nearest neighbors*—other users that had similar preferences to those of the active user in the past. In the next step, prediction for item i is computed based on the ratings for i made by other peer users. It assumes that user preferences remain stable and consistent over time.

3.2.1 Simple Example

Table 3.1 shows a database of ratings of the active user, i.e., Alice, and other users. The items were rated on a 1-to-5 scale, with "5" indicating a strong like. The task for recommender system, here, is to predict whether the active user—Alice will like or dislike "Item5", which has not been yet used or rated by Alice. To perform the prediction, the system has to find users similar to Alice, in the first place. In the second step, the system has to predict whether Alice will like or dislike the item based on ratings of similar users, found in the first step.

Similarity Measures

Different measures can be used to determine the set of similar users. The most common similarity measure used in recommendation systems is *Pearson's correlation coefficient* Eq. 3.1. Other similarity measures possible to use are: the simplest *Euclidean distance, the Minkowski distance* (a generalization of Euclidean distance), *the Mahalanobis distance, cosine similarity* or the *L2 norm*.

$$sim(a, b) = \frac{\Sigma_i (r_{a,i} - \bar{r}_a)(r_{b,i} - \bar{r}_b)}{\sqrt{\Sigma_i (r_{a,i} - \bar{r}_a)^2 \Sigma_i (r_{b,i} - \bar{r}_b)^2}} \tag{3.1}$$

The Pearson correlation coefficient takes values in range from $+1$ (strong positive correlation) to -1 (strong negative correlation). Similarity measure $sim(a, b)$ of users a and b, given the rating matrix R, is defined in formula Eq. 3.1. $r_{a,i}$ denotes rating of user a for the item i. $\bar{r}_a$ is average rating of user a. After computing this coefficient between Alice and each other user it turns out, that *User1* and *User2* were similar to *Alice* behavior in the past (correspondingly similarity measures of 0.85 and 0.7).

After choosing *peer users* of Alice, it is possible to compute a prediction for Alice's rating of *Item5*. One possible formula for prediction for the rating of user a for item i, that factors the relative proximity of the nearest neighbors N and a's average rating is given by Eq. 3.2.

$$pred(a, i) = \bar{r}_a + \frac{\Sigma_b sim(a, b) * (r_{b,i} - \bar{r}_b)}{\Sigma_b sim(a, b)} \qquad (3.2)$$

In the given example, the prediction for Alice's rating for *Item5* based on the nearest neighbors, *User1* and *User2* ratings would be:

$$4 + 1/(0.85 + 0.7) * (0.85 * (3 - 2.4) + 0.7 * (5 - 3.8)) = 4.87 \qquad (3.3)$$

Probabilistic Recommendation Approaches

Probability theory can also be exploited as another way of making a prediction about how a given user will rate a certain item. In this method, the prediction problem is treated as a *classification problem*, which means assigning an object to one of several predefined categories. One of standard technique in classification is based on *Bayes classifiers*. On the simple example presented above, the prediction task would be formulated as the problem of calculating the most probable rating value for *Item5*, given the set of Alice's other ratings and the ratings of the other users. In this method, *conditional probabilities* will be computed for each possible rating value, and then prediction will be selected as the one with the highest probability. Bayes theorem is used to compute posterior probability $P(Y|X)$ through the *class-conditional* probability $P(X|Y)$, the probability of Y and the probability of X (see formula Eq. 3.4). In the presented example, P(Y) might be a probability of a rating value 1 for *Item5* or any other possible rating value, and X being Alice's other ratings.

$$P(Y|X) = \frac{P(X|Y) * P(Y)}{P(X)} \qquad (3.4)$$

Under assumption that user ratings are *conditionally independent*, a *Naive Bayes* classifier can be built to compute posterior probability for each value of Y.

3.2.2 Example Applications

A real-world example of collaborative recommendation approach is the *Google News* personalization engine [JZFF10]. It presents news articles from thousands of sources, in a personalized way to signed-in users. The recommendation is based on the click history of the active user and the history of the larger community (with click being interpreted as a positive rating).

There have been many other collaborative systems developed in the academia and the industry. *Grundy* [AT05] was the first recommender system to model users by a mechanism called *stereotypes*, which are in turn used to build individual user models and recommend relevant books. *GroupLens*, *Video Recommender* and *Ringo* [AT05] were the first systems to use collaborative filtering algorithms to automate prediction. Other examples of collaborative recommender systems include the book recommendation system from *Amazon.com* and the *Jester* system that recommends jokes [AT05].

Collaborative Filtering in Medicine

Although collaborative recommenders are used mostly by commercial organizations to make predictions about user preferences for consumer items, many of the advantages offered by CF for the task of predicting user preferences are also relevant to the goal of assessing patients. Recently, studies employing collaborative techniques of RS in medical care have been conducted. Their motivation is to advise a consulting patient, based on the medical records of patients with similar indications. Collaborative filtering requires access to user profiles to identify user preferences and make recommendations.

To transfer the RS methodology to medical applications:

- patients are identified with *users*,
- patterns containing data of medical histories and physical examinations are identified with *user profiles*,
- a notion of *similarity* is employed for patients as it is for users,
- patient diagnoses are identified with *user ratings*.

Therefore, it is a logical development to employ recommender systems based on collaborative filtering to solve the medical problems.

The paper [HS10] presents a CF as a framework for clinical risk stratification. As CF finds similarities both between individual and items, the approach, presented in the paper, matched patients, as well as patient characteristics, to adverse outcomes (cardiovascular case). The approach translated to the following abstractions: predicting user ratings for items to predicting the risk of patients for adverse outcomes (risk to ratings; patients to users; patient characteristics as well as outcomes, to items). The approach in [HS10] assesses risk by comparing new patients to historical cases, and also by comparing the outcomes of interest to other outcomes or patient characteristics in the dataset (using information from neighboring patients and clinical attributes).

Though examples, as presented in the paper [HS10] exist, CF techniques are still applied to somehow narrowed range of domains: the most popular being movies and books, and many algorithms are improved only on such datasets.

3.3 Content-Based Recommendation

In the *content-based* approach, recommendation systems can be seen as tools to cope with information overload and stem from concepts such as information retrieval and information filtering. In discriminating between relevant and irrelevant items, they exploit information derived from the items' contents. They associate the derived content with the user profile or characteristic. The system learns to recommend items similar to those that the user liked in the past, so prediction is based on feature similarity between items (and not on similarity between users as in collaborative approach). In other words, systems implementing a content-based recommendation approach analyze a set of items' content previously rated by a user, and build a model or profile of user interests based on the features of the objects rated by that user [KRRS11]. Such approach makes recommender systems a way of personalizing their content for users or as user-modeling tools. Prediction is basically based on matching new item content with the attributes of the user profile.

3.3.1 High-Level Architecture

The three major components of content-based systems, as depicted in Fig. 3.3, are:

- *Content analyzer*—includes preprocessing step to extract structured information, feature extraction applied to data in order to shift item representation from the

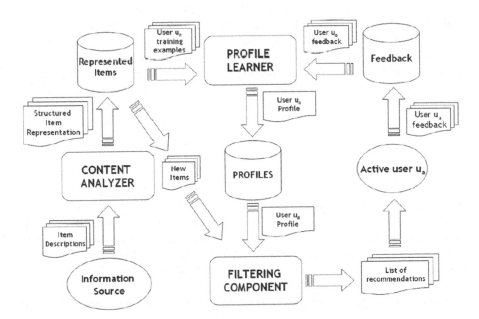

Fig. 3.3 High level architecture of a Content-based Recommender [KRRS11]

original information space to the target one, which is the input to the *Profile learner*,

- *Profile learner*—constructs the user profile based on generalization of the user preferences (through machine learning techniques),
- *Filtering component*—exploits the user profile to suggest relevant items, by matching the profile representation against that of items to be recommended.

Besides these components, there is a *Feedback* repository that stores the reactions (*annotations*) of a user to items, which are then used to update the *profile* of the active user u_a. The reactions are stored together with the related item descriptions, in order to be exploited during the process of learning a model useful to predict the relevance of newly presented items. User tastes usually change in time, so the up-to-date information must be provided to the *Profile Learner* in order to automatically update the user profile. The constant iteration of the feedback-learning cycle over time allows the system to consider the dynamic nature of user preferences.

3.3.2 Content Representation and Recommender Techniques

Content Representation

Items, often referred to as *documents*, can be described in the simplest way by an explicit list of *features*, also often called *attributes, characteristics*, or *item profiles*. For example, books can be described by characteristics such as title, genre, author, type, price, or keywords (and correspondingly, patients—by demographics, medical evaluation, etc.). Users should be asked to rate a set of items, either as a whole or along different dimensions. Based on this essential information, content-based recommendation systems evaluate how much a not-yet-seen item is "similar" to items the active user has liked in the past. Various similarity measures are feasible, depending on the problem area. The advanced technique of content-based representation is based on explicitly asking the user about their preferences, for instance, for a desired price range or a set of preferred genres, to weight the importance of certain attributes.

Boolean Vectors

As content-based systems were originally developed to filter and recommend text-based items such as e-mail messages or news, it is common to represent this type of items as a list of words that appear within the document. Such list can be encoded in different ways. It can be a list of all the words that appear in all documents, where "1" indicates that a word appears in a document, and "0"—that the word does not appear (boolean vector representation). Correspondingly, user profile can also be described by such a list and then matching can be done by measuring the overlap of interest and document content.

TF-IDF

Another way of describing document content, that takes into account frequency of words appearing in the document, is so called *TF-IDF* (*term frequency-inverse document frequency*). It additionally considers the length of the document (so that to prevent longer documents from getting a higher relevance weight). *Inverse document frequency* also reduces the weight of keywords that appear very often in all documents (because frequent words are not discriminating documents), so words that appear in only a few documents are given more weight. On the other hand, TF-IDF vectors are typically large and very sparse. Additional text preprocessing techniques can be used to reduce the dimensionality (for example removing stop words and stemming). *Feature selection*, a method of dimensionality reduction, is the process of choosing a subset of available terms, based on some statistical measures such as χ^2 (chi-squared) test.

Similarity-Based Retrieval

Similarity measures for vector-space documents are based on techniques such as:

- *nearest neighbors* (kNN),
- *relevance feedback* method, developed in the late 1960s by Rocchio for SMART system—a technique that helps users to incrementally refine queries based on previous search results.

Classification methods form the secondary category of the filtering component and include:

- probabilistic methods (Bayes classifiers),
- linear classifiers (for example support vector machines),
- decision trees (for example based on *ID3* or, the later, *C4.5* algorithm) and *random forests*,
- rule induction (similar to extracting decision rules, built, for example, on *RIPPER* algorithm).

The last method, based on rule induction has two advantages over other learning methods. First, the rules can serve as a basis for generating explanations for the system's recommendations. Second, existing prior domain knowledge can be incorporated in the models.

3.3.3 Example Applications

Considering industrial adoption, content-based systems are rarely found in commercial environments. Most of those successfully applied were developed in academic settings. In the area of *Web recommenders*, famous systems, in literature, are: *Letizia, Personal Web Watcher, Syskill & Webert, ifWeb, Amalthea* and *WebMate*. Other examples, for news filtering, are: *The Information Finder*, *Newsweeder*, *NewsRec*, *NewT*, *PSUN*, *INFOrmer*, *NewsDude*, *Daily Learner*, and *YourNews*.

Web Recommenders

Letizia is a web-browser extension that tracks the user's behavior and based on that, builds a personalized model. It also collects the user's feedback to infer the user's preferences. *Personal Web Watcher* is similar solution that learns user's behavior by tracking pages, they visit, and documents under those links, and one link further. Visited web-pages are processed as positive examples and non-visited as negative examples. *Amalthea* is a solution, which additionally implements agent technology, performing information filtering. *Syskill & Webert* system has web browsing assistants, which use past ratings to predict, whether user would be interested in the links on a web page. It represents documents with the most 128 words. *ifWeb* represents profiles in the form of a weighted semantic network.

News Filtering

In the field of news filtering, in solutions such as *NewT*, there are several agents, each for different kind of information, e.g. one for political news, one for sports, etc. It also allows users to provide positive or negative feedback on articles, authors or sources. Another system—*NewsDude* learns short- and long-term profiles. The former is based on TF-IDF representation and cosine similarity measure, the latter—on naive Bayes classifier. A similar approach, of such two models, is *Daily Learner*, a learning agent for wireless information access. In this case the short-term model is learned with nearest neighbors text classification algorithm, while the long-term collects long-term interests of users and is based on naive Bayes classifier. More advanced representation of documents is implemented in systems *PSUN* and *INFOrmer*. The first represents articles so that recurring words are recorded by means of *n-grams*, stored in a network of mutually attracting or repelling words. In addition, users have multiple profiles competing via a genetic algorithm. *INFOrmer* uses a semantic network for both user profile and article representation.

Books, Movies and Music Recommendation

Content-based recommendation exist also for a number of different application areas. *LIBRA* recommends books, exploiting descriptions on Amazon on-line digital store, by means of a naive Bayes text categorization. *Citeseer* assists users with searching for a scientific literature. It exploits common citations in the papers. *INTIMATE* is a system for movie recommendation, which uses text categorization techniques based on information retrieved from the Internet Movie Database. The users of this system are asked to explicitly provide ratings for movies. In the application area of music recommendations, the most notable content-based system is *Pandora* that exploits manual descriptions. Many recommendation systems in this application area are however collaborative-based.

Ontology-Based Systems

Besides solutions presented above, which are mainly based on keyword representation for both items and profiles, it is also possible to infuse knowledge by means of ontologies and encyclopedic knowledge sources. Ontology-based representation allows to add some "intelligence" and ability to interpret natural language. *SiteIF*, for example, is a personal agent for multilingual news Web site, with a representation process based on external knowledge source—MultiWordNet (multilingual lexical database, where different language senses are aligned). In *ITR (ITem Recommender)*, which provides recommendations in several domains (e.g., movies, music, books), linguistic knowledge about items' descriptions comes from the WordNet lexical ontology. *SEWeP (Semantic Enhancement for Web Personalization)*, a Web personalization system, uses logs and the semantics of a Website's content, and also WordNet to "interpret" the content of an item by using word sense disambiguation. *Quickstep*, a system for the recommendation of on-line academic research papers, adopts a research paper topic ontology based on the computer science classifications. The process of learning can also benefit from the infusion of exogenous knowledge (externally supplied). Examples of general-purpose knowledge databases are: Open Directory Project (ODP), Yahoo! Web Directory, and Wikipedia.

Healthcare

The paper [WP14] claims, that content-based approach is suitable for the purpose of building *Health Recommender Systems*. It also argues that collaborative approach is unsuitable, because it inspects user profiles *across users*, which would incur too high security risk (personal health data has to be kept confidential). The solution proposed in [WP14] leverages information of a graph data structure related to health concepts derived from *Wikipedia* to compute individual relevance.

Another example is *Personal Health Explorer*, proposed by Morrell and Kerschberg (2012), a semantic health recommendation system that uses an agent based framework to retrieve content from web resources related to individual's personal health records.

A basic form of content recommendation is also provided by consumer-centric web portals for medical information, for example, symptoms and diseases. If a user of such web portal has an account and a medical profile (that is, a health record) linked to it, RS can provide matching health information of high individual relevance. However, such systems are aimed at ordinary people, so-called "laymen", rather than at medical personnel.

3.4   Knowledge-Based Recommendation

When a system needs to exploit additional knowledge to generate recommendations, a *knowledge-based* approach is needed. Such knowledge may be elicited interactively by interacting with the user. Sometimes there is confusion in differentiating between content- and knowledge-based systems. Content-based systems typically work on text documents or other items, for which features can be automatically extracted, and for which some learning method is applied. In contrast, knowledge-based systems rely mostly on externally provided information about items.

Knowledge-based approach is advantageous, in scenarios, where collaborative filtering or content-based approaches show limitations. For example, buying a house, a car, or a computer is not a frequently made decision. Pure CF system would not perform well, because of the low number of available ratings. For content-based systems the time span between ratings would make them useless (for example five-year-old ratings for computers would be rather inappropriate). Also, preferences evolve over time. In the case when requirements for an item formulated by user are set explicitly, they are not easily incorporated into collaborative- or content-based frameworks. The main drawback of knowledge-based systems is a need for knowledge acquisition—a common bottleneck for many artificial intelligence applications.

The most common division of knowledge-based systems is that between *constraint-based* systems and *case-based* systems. The recommendation process in both types looks similar: the requirements are elicited from the user and then solution is identified by the system. If the solution is not found, however, the requirements must be changed by the user. Optionally, explanation for the recommendation may also be provided to the user. The difference between constraint- and cased-based systems lies in the way the provided knowledge is used: the former rely on an explicitly defined set of recommendation rules, whereas the latter retrieve the items that are similar, based on various measures.

3.4.1   Knowledge Representation and Reasoning

Detailed knowledge about items is pivotal for knowledge-based systems. Based on item feature values and requirements defined by the user, which are expressed as desired values or value ranges for an item feature, selecting the right item is the task of recommendation problem. A constraint-based recommendation problem can be represented as a *constraint satisfaction problem*, which can be solved by a constraint solver or as a query by a database engine. Case-based systems rely mostly on similarity metrics to select the desired items (for example, so called *distance similarity*). Constraint-based systems can exploit the mechanism of a *recommender knowledge base*. If the problem is unsatisfiable, the constraints can be relaxed until a corresponding solution is found.

It is also important to rank recommended items according to their utility for the user. Each item is evaluated according to a predefined set of dimensions that provide an aggregated view on the basic item properties.

3.4.2 Example Applications

Constraint-Based

One of the commercial developed examples of constraint-based recommender system is VITA financial services application for Hungarian financial service provider [FISZ07]. VITA supports sales representatives in sales dialogs with customers. Such representatives are challenged by the increased complexity of service solutions, they do not know how to recommend such services. The goal of developing a system supporting sales representatives was to increase their overall productivity and advisory quality in sales dialogs.

Figure 3.4 shows architecture of the VITA sales support environment [JZFF10].

The functionality of VITA system was deployed on a web server application and was available for both sales representatives at office and external sales agents preparing and conducting sales dialogs, and some functionality is provided for sales representatives using their own laptops. Thus, new versions of sales dialogs and

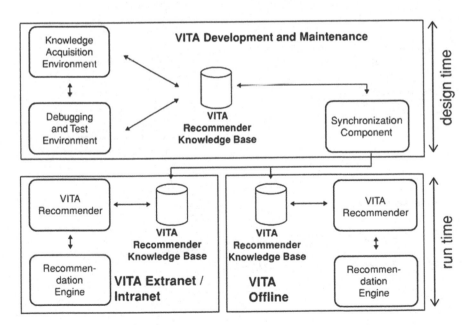

Fig. 3.4 VITA sales support environment [FISZ07]

knowledge bases are automatically installed when the sales representative is connected with the intranet. Such solution helps in dealing with highly complex and frequently changing recommendation knowledge bases. Also, automated testing and debugging of knowledge bases was implemented into the solution.

The knowledge base of VITA system consists of the following elements:

- *Customer properties*—requirements articulated by each customer,
- *Product properties and instances*—predefined properties of each product,
- *Constraints*—restrictions defining which products should be recommended in which context,
- *Advisory process definition*—definitions of sales dialogs.

A recommendation process in the system is divided into a number of steps (see Fig. 3.5): *requirements elicitation, creditworthiness check, product advisory/ selection*, and *detailed calculation/result presentation*.

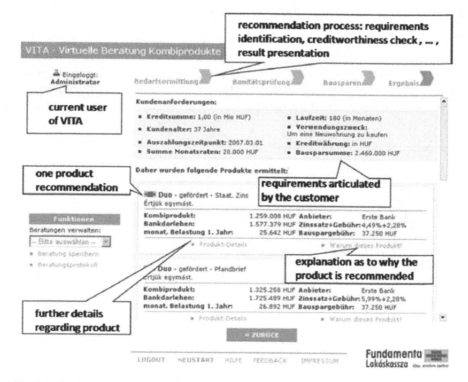

Fig. 3.5 Screen of sales support system—VITA [FISZ07]

Case-Based

Example of case-based knowledge system would be *Entree*—a system recommending restaurants in Chicago, which uses some domain knowledge about restaurants, cuisines, and foods. User interaction is conducted via web-based interface—users enter their preferences and requirements. The system cycles through several iterations of recommendations. At each cycle, it retrieves a set of candidate items from the item database that fulfills the criteria defined by the user, and sorts them according to their similarity to the currently recommended item. The most similar are then returned.

Some knowledge-based recommendation systems have been developed for application domains where domain knowledge is readily available in some structured machine-readable form, for example, as an ontology. Examples of such approach are *Qiuickstep* and *Foxtrot* systems, which use research paper topic ontology to recommend online research articles to the users.

3.5 Hybrid Recommender Systems

Pure content-based recommender systems proved to have some limitations, which led to the development of hybrid systems that combine the advantages of different recommendation techniques. As hybrid recommender system, can be understood any combination of the above-mentioned techniques. Combination can be any of the following [AT05]:

- combining separate recommender systems—either combining ratings obtained from them individually or using the output that is "better" than others at a given moment,
- adding characteristics of one approach to another model,
- developing a single unifying recommendation model—for example, using content-based and collaborative characteristics in a single rule-based classifier.

3.5.1 Example Applications

Hybrid approaches demonstrated to provide more accurate recommendations than pure approaches [AT05]. Real-world examples of systems that combine collaborative and content-based methods are: *Fab, WebWatcher, P-Tango, ProfBuilder, PTV, Content-boosted Collaborative Filtering, CinemaScreen. Fab* is based on traditional collaborative techniques, but also maintains the content-based profiles for each user. These content-based profiles are used to calculate the similarity between two users [AT05].

3.6 Discussion

Considering the decision problem that should be solved by a recommender system in this work (tinnitus characterization and treatment) and the given dataset's characteristics, it is argued that neither pure collaborative approach nor pure content-based approach would be effective to use. On the other hand, rule-based approach could be more convenient and appropriate, as extraneous knowledge base is provided. Rules could model the complex human expert behavior and decision-making.

Considering the first discussed approach—collaborative filtering, it would be difficult to represent patients' data as a simple item rating matrix. The items (treatment methods) are not explicitly specified (treatment is complex and multi-factorial) and have to be extracted first. It is impossible to obtain item ratings (that is a recovery rate) for each of them for each patient (resulting matrix would be very sparse). This is because, patient is treated with one method only at a given time, alternatively other methods are applied later, but then, the patient's medical conditions change (temporal dependencies have to be considered). In other words, the treatment process is not repeatable, as in case of buying books or CDs. The decision process in medical evaluation is much more complex, rather unique and highly personalized than very frequent and common buying decisions (of books, CDs, etc.). Thus, it cannot be expressed as easily as preference rating given by the users of an online bookstore, for example. Furthermore, the size of dataset is not large enough (about 550 patients) to find users similar to the one under consideration (this problem is known as *startup problem*). For these reasons and given the specific knowledge domain (protocol of TRT treatment), *collaborative filtering* would be less suitable approach for a RS for tinnitus.

Secondly, as already mentioned in the section about content-based recommendation, RS solutions for medicine based on this approach are developed for supporting "laymen" and Internet users, seeking information about medical conditions, rather than supporting medical professional in highly specialized decision-making. Content-based approach, similarly to collaborative approach, has a drawback of so called "new user problem", that is, enough ratings have to be collected before such RS can really understand "user preferences" and provide accurate recommendations. This approach would not be suitable, as there are not many "item ratings", that is tinnitus treatment results, for a one given patient (the same as it is unsuitable for infrequent buying decisions—cars or house). Moreover, the solution for tinnitus treatment of a given patient should take into account successful treatment methods applied to other patients, while content-based approach focuses only on "preferences" (medical condition) of one particular "user" (patient). Content-based approach is also known for its tendency to suffer from overspecialization, that is, inability for finding something unexpected, and the tendency to produce recommendations with a limited degree of novelty.

With all these disadvantages, however, some content retrieval techniques might be used for exploring medical documents and data from a patient's personal health records that are unstructured (data entries of medical records are frequently stored as unstructured plain text—discharge letters, descriptions of diagnoses, etc.). Content-based approach could be used for retrieving information from textual information of tinnitus databases, such as treatment progress descriptions.

To sum up, traditional recommendation approaches (content-based filtering and collaborative filtering) are well-suited for the recommendation of "quality and taste" products, such as books, movies, or news. As already indicated above, these approaches are not the best choice in the context of products such as cars, computers, apartments, financial or medical services (where decision is rather one-off than frequent). Knowledge-based recommender technologies help to tackle these challenges, by exploiting explicit user requirements (patient's characteristic) and deep knowledge about the underlying problem domain for the calculation of recommendations.

Tinnitus treatment is a decision problem that requires some *domain knowledge*. Therefore, approach proposed within this book is knowledge-based recommendation, with the domain knowledge specified in the form of rules, automatically extracted from the given dataset. This approach also does not require large amount of data and there is no *cold start* problem (since requirements are directly elicited within a recommendation session). It allows to specify a particular user's (patient's) needs or interests (medical conditions). The alternative approach for tinnitus diagnosis and treatment could be also a hybrid approach combining collaborative filtering and knowledge based models, depending on dataset size, and possible extension of information-retrieval feature to explore textual descriptions or comments on treatment methods.

The next chapter describes the chosen approach, based on rules and knowledge extraction, in greater detail.

Chapter 4
Knowledge Discovery Approach for Recommendation

Abstract This chapter presents concepts of action rules, proposed by Ras and Wieczorkowska in 2000 [RW00] and meta-actions, as a proposed approach for building a rule-based (knowledge-based) recommender system for tinnitus treatment, and motivation for using such methods. It also presents theoretical foundations and algorithms for automatic action rules extraction, as methods for domain knowledge discovery.

4.1 Basic Concepts

Approach based on actions presents a new way in machine learning, which solves problems that traditional methods, such as classification or association rules, cannot handle. Its purpose is to analyze data to improve understanding of it and seek specific actions (recommendations) to enhance the decision-making process. In contrast to association rule learning (Agrawal et al. 1993), action rule approaches mine actionable patterns that can be employed to reach a desired goal, instead of only extracting passive relations between variables. Since its introduction in 2000, action rules have been successfully applied in many domain areas including business [RW00]), medical diagnosis and treatment (Wasyluk et al. 2008; Zhang et al. 2010), and music automatic indexing and retrieval (Ras and Wieczorkowska 2010; Ras and Dardzinska 2011).

An *action rule* is defined as "a rule extracted from an information system that describes a possible transition of objects from one state to another with respect to a distinguished attribute called a decision attribute" [Ras15]. To understand this definition, it is important to introduce some associated concepts, which will be explained later. Action rules can be further improved by the introduction of *meta-actions* that help control the actions. Meta-actions are mechanism used to acquire knowledge about possible transitions in the information systems and their causes. This knowledge is then used in triggering particular action rules, in order to move objects fromtheir current state to a more desirable state. Meta-actions were first introduced

© Springer International Publishing AG 2017   35
K.A. Tarnowska et al., *Decision Support System for Diagnosis and Treatment of Hearing Disorders*, Studies in Computational Intelligence 685,
DOI 10.1007/978-3-319-51463-5_4

to mine actionable patterns, then formally defined and used to discover action rules based on tree classifiers Ras [RD09]. They were also used to personalize action rules based on patients' side-effects in [TKHR13].

Action rules seem to be especially promising in the field of medical data, as a doctor can examine the effect of treatment decisions on a patient's improved state [Tho11]. For example, in the tinnitus dataset, such indicator of tracking improvement progress would be *total score* attribute, calculated as sum of Newman form (Tinnitus Handicap Inventory—see Appendix C) responses. Meta-actions would, on the other hand, represent treatments, prescribed by doctors to their patients (in tinnitus case—counseling, instrumentation and their fitting). Meta-actions, in the context of the healthcare, represent the patient's state transition from an initial state to a different state. Action rules would be used to move a patient from the sick population state to the healthy population state.

4.1.1　Information Systems

A concept of *Information System* stems from the theory of rough sets, developed by Zdzislaw Pawlak at the beginning of 1980s [PM81]. Back then, it was a novel approach to the formal representation of knowledge description, especially of knowledge that was given incompletely and/or imprecisely. Since its introduction, the theory of rough sets was developing extensively all around the word, and especially in Poland. Application of rough sets theory in machine learning, image recognition, control of technological processes and expert systems confirmed its usefulness in practical settings.

The rough set theory handles data analysis organized in the form of tables. The data may come from experts, measurements or tests. The main goals of the data analysis is a retrieval of interesting and novel patterns, associations, more precise problem analysis, as well as designing a tool for automatic data classification.

Definition 4.1 An *Information System* is defined as a pair $S = (U, A)$, where U is a nonempty, finite set, called *the universe*, and A is a nonempty, finite set of attributes i.e. $a : U \rightarrow V_a$ for $a \in A$, where V_a is called the domain of a [RW00].

Elements of U are called *objects*. A special case of *Information Systems* is called a *Decision Table* [Paw85].

4.1.2　Decision Tables

In a decision table, some attributes are called *conditions* and the others are called *decisions*. In many practical applications, decision is a singleton set. Figure 4.1 depicts a decision table with 8 objects describing patients with 3 attributes: *Headache, Muscle*

U	Headache	Muscle pain	Temp.	Flu
p1	Yes	Yes	Normal	No
p2	Yes	Yes	High	Yes
p3	Yes	Yes	Very-high	Yes
p4	No	Yes	Normal	No
p5	No	No	High	No
p6	No	Yes	Very-high	Yes
p7	No	Yes	High	Yes
p8	No	No	Very-high	No

Fig. 4.1 Example of a decision table with patients' data

Patient	Age	Sex	Chol.	Resting ECG	Heart rate	Sick
p_1	53	M	203	hyp	155	yes
p_2	60	M	185	hyp	155	yes
p_3	40	M	199	norm	178	no
p_4	46	F	243	norm	144	no
p_5	62	F	294	norm	162	no
p_6	43	M	177	hyp	120	yes
p_7	76	F	197	abnorm	116	no
p_8	62	M	267	norm	99	yes
p_9	57	M	274	norm	88	yes
p_{10}	72	M	200	abnorm	100	no

Fig. 4.2 Another example of a decision table with patients' data

pain and *Temperature*. Decision is a binary attribute specifying if a patient has a flu or not.

Based on knowledge represented in a form of a decision table, it is possible to model and simulate decision-making processes. The knowledge in a decision table is represented by associating or identifying decision values with some values of conditional attributes. In practical settings, decision tables are created from ordinary tables or database, by specifying conditions and decisions. Conditional attributes are characteristics that are easily available, for example measurements, parameters, personal data, etc. Decision is a feature related to not commonly known knowledge, for example given by an expert (doctor for instance) or based on later observations (for example—stock exchange rating). Decision is known only for the objects from the training table. The goal is to use it for establishing a decision for new objects, based on their attributes.

In a dataset, presented in Fig. 4.2, decision attribute would be similar as in Table in Fig. 4.1—whether a person is sick or not. In tinnitus dataset—a decision attribute would be patient's category, with values in the range of 0–4 (see Table 2.1). This attribute would classify objects (patients) into tinnitus treatment group, taking into account medical/audiological evaluation and form responses.

For action rules extraction, it is also relevant to differentiate between so-called *flexible* attributes, which can be changed, and *stable* attributes [RW00], which cannot be changed: $A = A_{St} \cup A_{Fl}$, where A_{St} and A_{Fl} denote *stable* attributes and *flexible* attributes respectively. Example of a stable attribute in medical data would be *Gender*, *Age*, while flexible might be *Cholesterol level* or *Hearing Device*.

4.1.3   Reducts

In decision systems not every attribute in the database is necessary for decision-making process. The goal is to choose some subset of attributes essential for this. It leads to definition of *reducts*, that is, minimal subsets of attributes that keep the characteristics of the full dataset. In the context of action rule discovery an *action reduct* is a minimal set of attribute values distinguishing a favorable object from another. Before defining formally a *reduct*, it is necessary to introduce a *discernibility relation*.

Definition 4.2 Let objects $x, y \in U$ and set of attributes $B \subset A$. We say that x, y are *discernible* by B when there exists $a \in B$ such that $a(x) \neq b(y)$. x, y are *indiscernible* by B when they are identical on B, that is, $a(x) = b(y)$ for each $a \in B$. $[x]_B$ denotes a set of objects indiscernible with x by B.

Furthermore, following statements are true:

- for each objects x, y either $[x]_B = [y]_B$ or $[x]_B \cap [y]_B = \emptyset$,
- *indiscernibility relation* is an equivalence relation,
- each set of attributes $A \subset B$ determines a partition of a set of objects into disjoint subsets.

Example 4.1 In the table presented in Fig. 4.1 objects p_1, p_2, p_3 are indiscernible for attribute subset $B = \{Headache, Musclepain\}$, and in the Table 4.2 objects p_1, p_2 are indiscernible for attributes $B = \{RestingECG, Heartrate\}$. Also, in the first case, there are three disjoint indiscernibility classes:

- $[p_1]_B = \{p_1, p_2, p_3\}$,
- $[p_4]_B = \{p_4, p_6, p_7\}$,
- $[p_5]_B = \{p_5, p_8\}$.

In the second table, we can see the need to discretize some numerical values, because the search for the same attribute values is very unlikely to succeed (that two the same real numbers are found). The numerical values are, then, replaced by the value representing an interval, to which an original value belongs.

Definition 4.3 A set of attributes $B \subset A$ is called *reduct of the decision table* if and only if:

- B keeps the discernibility of A, that is, for each $x, y \in U$, if x, y are discernible by A, then they are also discernible by B,

- *B* is irreducible, that is, none of its proper subset keeps discernibility properties of *A* (that is, *B* is minimal in terms of discernibility).

The set of attributes appearing in every reduct of information system *A* (decision table *DT*) is called *the core*.

4.2 Decision Rules

Decision rule, for a given decision table, is a rule in the form: $(\phi \rightarrow \delta)$, where ϕ is called *antecedent* (or *assumption*) and δ is called *descendant* (or *thesis*) of the rule. The antecedent for an atomic rule can be a single term or a conjunction of *k* elementary conditions: $\phi = p_1 \wedge p_2 \wedge \cdots \wedge p_n$, and δ is a decision attribute. Decision rule describing a class K_j means that objects, which satisfy (match) the rule's antecedent, belong to K_j.

Each rule can be characterized by the following features:

- length(r) = number of descriptors in the antecedent of the rule,
- [r] = a set of objects from *U* matching the rule's antecedent,
- support(r) = number of objects from *U* matching the rule's antecedent: $\|[r]\|$ (relative support is further divided by number of objects *N*),
- confidence(r) = reliability of the rule: $\dfrac{|[r] \cap DEC_k|}{|[r]|}$-number of objects matching both rule's antecedent and descendant, divided by absolute support.

The problem of finding a minimal set of rules that fully describes the dataset (covers all samples from dataset) and then classifies them correctly is a NP-problem. A transformation of such problem into a problem of minimum coverage of a set is used for proofs.

On the grounds of rough sets theory, reducts are used in algorithms generating all decision rules from the given decision table. The algorithm uses relative reducts for each object belonging to the *U*. Boolean logic and inference are often applied in such algorithms, based on construction of so-called *discernibility matrix* and transformations of *discernibility functions*, which are derived from such matrix. A set of *prime implicants* of these functions are then used for a generation of *global (relative) reducts* or *local (relative) reducts* associated with singular objects. Rules for a given decision class are then generated from reducts. Besides such algorithms, finding reducts exactly, there are methods based on approximation algorithms, genetic algorithms, for example.

4.3   Classification Rules

In the context of prediction problem, decision rules generated from training dataset, are used for classifying new objects (for example classifying a new patient for tinnitus category). New objects are understood as objects that were not used for the rules induction (new patients coming to the doctor). The new objects are described by attribute values (for instance a patient with conducted audiological evaluation and form responses). The goal of classification is to assign a new object to one of the decision classes. Prediction is performed by matching the object description with the rule antecedents. Furthermore, if the original value of decision class is known for this object, it is called a *testing sample*, because it can be used to compare the true with the predicted class label.

After finding a set of decision rules, it is possible to find a description of decision classes and classify objects based on that. Classification rules are generated from decision rules by the following procedure:

- training phase: a set of rules *RULES(A)* is generated from the given decision table *A*,
- selection phase: *RULES(A)* is searched for rules matching object x. These rules are denoted as *MatchRules(A,x)*,
- classification phase: decision class is allocated for x, with the use of rules from *MatchRules(A,x)*, according to the following schema:

  - if *MatchRules(A,x)* is empty, the decision for x is *UNKNOWN*,
  - if *MatchRules(A,x)* contains only objects from decision class k, then $dec(x) = k$,
  - if *MatchRules(A,x)* contains objects from different decision classes, then decision for x is determined by some chosen voting schema amongst rules from *MatchRules(A,x)*.

The set of rules should be filtered in many possible ways, in order to obtain best rules to be used by the classifier. Classification trees are also used to generate classification rules.

4.4   Action Rules

An *action* is understood as a way of controlling or changing some of attribute values in an information system to achieve desired results [IRT11]. An *action rule* is defined [RW00] as a rule extracted from an information system, that describes a transition that may occur within objects from one state to another, with respect to decision attribute, as defined by the user. In nomenclature, action rule is defined as a term: $[(\omega) \wedge (\alpha \rightarrow \beta) \rightarrow (\Phi \rightarrow \Psi)]$, where ω denotes conjunction of fixed condition attributes, $(\alpha \rightarrow \beta)$ are proposed changes in values of flexible features, and $(\Phi \rightarrow \Psi)$ is a desired change of decision attribute (action effect) [Ras15]. Action rule discovery applied to tinnitus dataset could, for example, suggest a change in a flexible attribute, such as type of instrument, to help "reclassify" or "transit" an object (patient) to a different category (less severe) and consequently, attain better treatment effectiveness.

4.4.1 Definitions

An action rule is built from *atomic action sets*.

Definition 4.4 *Atomic action term* is an expression $(a, a_1 \rightarrow a_2)$, where a is attribute, and $a_1, a_2 \in V_a$, where V_a is a domain of attribute a.

If $a_1 = a_2$ then a is called stable on a_1.

Definition 4.5 By *action sets* we mean the smallest collection of sets such that:

1. If t is an atomic action term, then t is an action set.
2. If t_1, t_2 are action sets, then $t_1 \wedge t_2$ is a candidate action set.
3. If t is a candidate action set and for any two atomic actions $(a, a_1 \rightarrow a_2), (b, b_1 \rightarrow b_2)$ contained in t we have $a \neq b$, then t is an action set. Here b is another attribute $(b \in A)$, and $b_1, b_2 \in V_b$.

Definition 4.6 By an *action rule* we mean any expression $r = [t_1 \Rightarrow t_2]$, where t_1 and t_2 are action sets.

The interpretation of the action rule r is, that by applying the action set t_1, we would get, as a result, the changes of states in action set t_2.

Example 4.2 [KDJR14] Assuming that a, b and d are stable attribute, flexible attribute and decision attribute respectively in S, expressions (a, a_2), $(b, b_1 \rightarrow b_2)$, $(d, d_1 \rightarrow d_2)$ are examples of atomic action sets. Expression (a, a_2) means that the value a_2 of attribute a remains unchanged, $(b, b_1 \rightarrow b_2)$ that value of attribute b is changed from b_1 to b_2. Expression $r = [\{(a, a_2) \wedge (b, b_1 \rightarrow b_2)\} \Rightarrow \{(d, d_1 \rightarrow d_2)\}]$ is an example of an action rule meaning that if value a_2 of a remains unchanged and value of b will change from b_1 to b_2, then the value of d will be expected to transition from d_1 to d_2. Rule r can be also perceived as the composition of two association rules r_1 and r_2, where $r_1 = [\{a, a_2) \wedge (b, b_1)\} \Rightarrow (d, d_1)]$ and $r_2 = [\{a, a_2) \wedge (b, b_2)\} \Rightarrow (d, d_2)]$.

Observation from the above example is that if the goal is to move patients having tinnitus from higher to lower severity group, we should find characteristics or methods of treatment for the patients or visits that have decision attribute d belonging to the class we aim for the treatment as a result. Therefore, using the theoretical example above, for the treated patient we should find another object (visit or patient) that have the same values for some stable attributes a (the same preconditions), but belong to lower tinnitus severity group (d_2 should be lower than d_1), and find atomic actions such as $(b, b_1 \rightarrow b_2)$ meaning that if changing the method of treatment for the first patient from b_1 to b_2, the expected recovery would be from category d_1 to d_2.

4.4.2 Algorithms

Action rules discovery is divided into two types [Ras15]:

- rule-based—prior extraction of classification rules is needed, actionable patterns are built on the foundations of pre-existing rules (for example DEAR algorithm),
- object-based—action rules are extracted directly from the database (for example ARED algorithm, similar to Apriori) [RDTW08].

In rule-based approach, action rules are built from certain pairs of classification rules. This approach is characterized by two main steps: (1) in the first step, a standard learning method is used to detect interesting patterns in the form of classification rules and (2) the second step is to use an automatic or semiautomatic strategy to inspect these rules and from their certain pairs derive possible action strategies.

In object-based approach, action rules are extracted directly from a dataset. The interpretation of object-driven action rules was first proposed by Hajja, Wieczorkowska, Ras, and Gubrynowicz in 2012. They showed that such rules can be applied for complex datasets, for example, containing various instances for the same object, and a temporal aspect coupled with each instance (as in case of tinnitus dataset). As a matter of fact, datasets with such structure can be frequently found in medical data, where for each unique patient, representing an object, multiple visits are recorded, and where in each visit (representing an instance) a timestamp is associated with the instance.

ARED—Action Rule Extraction from Decision Table
The following paragraph will present a method to construct action rules from a decision table containing both stable and flexible attributes. Presented ARED (Action Rule Extraction from Decision Table) algorithm [IR08] is based on Pawlak's model of an information system S. It uses a bottom-up approach to generate action rules having minimal attribute involvement, without the need to find classification rules in the first place. The goal in the algorithm, which is similar to Apriori, is to identify certain relationships between *granules*, defined by the indiscernibility relation on objects in S. Some of these relationships uniquely define action rules for S.

We assume that the decision attribute is d, stable attributes $A_{St} = \{a\}$, and the flexible attributes $A_{Fl} = \{b, c\}$, given the decision table as in Table 4.1. We also assume that the minimum support (λ_1) and confidence (λ_2) are given as 1 and 0.85.

The first step in the procedure is to find pessimistic interpretation in S of all attribute values in V, called *granules*. The granule a_1^*, associated with attribute value a_1 in S, is the set of objects having property a_1 (that is, objects $\{x_1, x_6, x_7, x_8\}$). The set of granules in a given S for attributes a, b, c is as follows:

$$a_1^* = \{x_1, x_6, x_7, x_8\}$$
$$a_2^* = \{x_2, x_3, x_4, x_5\}$$
$$b_1^* = \{x_1, x_2, x_4, x_6\}$$
$$b_2^* = \{x_7, x_8\}$$
$$b_3^* = \{x_5\}$$
$$c_1^* = \{x_1, x_4, x_8\}$$

Table 4.1 Decision table S
[IR08]

	a	b	c	d
x_1	a_1	b_1	c_1	d_1
x_2	a_2	b_1	c_2	d_1
x_3	a_2		c_2	d_1
x_4	a_2	b_1	c_1	d_1
x_5	a_2	b_3	c_2	d_1
x_6	a_1	b_1		d_2
x_7	a_1	b_2	c_2	d_1
x_8	a_1	b_2	c_1	d_3

$c_2^* = \{x_2, x_3, x_5, x_7\}$
and for the decision attribute:
$d_1^* = \{x_1, x_2, x_3, x_4, x_5, x_7\}$
$d_2^* = \{x_6\}$
$d_3^* = \{x_5\}$
The next step in the procedure is to find possible *property transitions* between objects in S. Let define two sets, τ and δ, such that:

- $\tau = T \wedge d_1$, where $d_1 \in V_d$, and $(\forall \rho_1 \in T \wedge d_1)(sup(\rho_1 \geq \lambda_1))$.
- $\delta = T \wedge d_2$, where $d_2 \in V_d$, and $(\forall \rho_2 \in T \wedge d_2)(sup(\rho_2 \geq \lambda_1))$.

T is a set of proper conjuncts built from elements in $\cup\{V_i, i \neq d, i \in A\}$. Proper conjunct is the one that contains maximum one element from each V_i. By $T \wedge d_i$, we mean $\{t \wedge d_i : t \in T\}$, $i = 1, 2$. The support of ρ_i, $sup(\rho_i)$ means the number of objects in S supporting all attribute values listed in ρ_i, $i = 1, 2$. This can be easily calculated by intersecting two granules: one for a conditional attribute and the second for the decision attribute: for example, $(a_1 \wedge d_2)^* = \{x_1, x_6, x_7, x_8\} \cap \{x_6\}$, $sup((a_1 \wedge d_2)^*) = 1$.

Such sets represent a relationship between conditional attributes and the decision attribute and property of a set of objects. If the property transition from τ to δ is valid, τ to δ are interpreted as the *condition* and the *decision* of an *action rule*.

ARED attempts to discover the shortest action rules in terms of the number of attributes, then iteratively generates longer action rules. Thus, firstly τ containing two elements is constructed, but only such that fulfill support criteria (Table 4.2).

In the next step, given τ and δ as in Table 4.2, we construct action rules by evaluating the validity of their transitions. All pairs from τ and δ are generated (if decision is equal the pair is omitted). There should also exist different flexible attribute values and be from the same domain. For example, $d_1 \neq d_2$ and $a_1 \neq a_2$ for $(a_1 \wedge d_2)^*$ and $(a_2 \wedge d_1)^*$, but because a is a stable attribute, no action rule is constructed. If two sets do not meet this condition, they are put in two separate arrays and are used to generate τ and δ for the next iteration (Table 4.4). For example, $(a_1 \wedge b_1 \wedge d_1) \implies (a_1 \wedge b_2 \wedge d_3)$ will be an action rule produced later. While producing action rules $\tau_i \implies \delta_1$ the condition for confidence is also checked (should be grater or equal λ_2

Table 4.2 2-Element τ and δ
[IR08]

τ	δ
$(a_1 \wedge d_1)$	$(a_1 \wedge d_1)$
$(a_1 \wedge d_2)$	$(a_1 \wedge d_2)$
$(a_1 \wedge d_3)$	$(a_1 \wedge d_3)$
$(a_2 \wedge d_1)$	$(a_2 \wedge d_1)$
$(b_1 \wedge d_1)$	$(b_1 \wedge d_1)$
$(b_1 \wedge d_2)$	$(b_1 \wedge d_2)$
$(b_2 \wedge d_1)$	$(b_2 \wedge d_1)$
$(b_2 \wedge d_3)$	$(b_2 \wedge d_3)$
$(b_3 \wedge d_1)$	$(b_3 \wedge d_1)$
$(c_1 \wedge d_1)$	$(c_1 \wedge d_1)$
$(c_1 \wedge d_3)$	$(c_1 \wedge d_3)$
$(c_2 \wedge d_1)$	$(c_2 \wedge d_1)$

to become an action rule). Confidence of $ar = \tau \implies \delta$ is computed using support of ar, which is the minimum of $(sup(\tau), sup(\delta))$:

$$conf(ar) = \frac{sup(ar)}{sup(\tau)}$$

Two-element action rules exacted from S are shown in Table 4.3. For example, $(b_1 \wedge d_2) \implies (b_2 \wedge d_1)$ is an action rule, and it is interpreted as, "if b changes from b_1 to b_2, then d changes from d_1 to d_2". If the confidence of a 2-element action rule is less than λ_2 (such as in two first in Table 4.4), however, the current τ_i and δ_j are considered in the next iteration of generating 3-element candidate sets (Table 4.5).

To find the action rules of length 3, we generate τ of length 3 from τs in Table 4.4. Two terms $\tau_1 = t_1 \wedge d_1$ and $\tau_2 = t_2 \wedge d_2$ are concatenated if $d_1 = d_2$ and $|t_1 \cup t_2| - |t_2 \cap t_1| = \{v_1 \in V_a, v_2 \in V_b\}$, where $a \neq b$. The set $\{\delta\}$ is generated from δs in Table 4.4 with the use of the same method. Therefore, they are generated independently. Table 4.5 shows those 3-element candidate sets. Corresponding action rule and invalid transitions are shown in Tables 4.6 and 4.7.

In the next iteration, we build an action rule with 4 elements (Table 4.8) from corresponding τ and δ. However, the generated rule is not included in the list of action rules, because its τ and δ are supersets of $(b_1 \wedge c_3 \wedge d_1) \implies (b_2 \wedge c_2 \wedge d_3)$, which is a more general action rule.

Then the process stops because there are no sets to be combined. The presented algorithm generates a complete set of shortest action rules.

Temporal constraints and object-driven assumptions

When dealing with particular datasets, which, for example, represent patients and visits, some constraints should be imposed on the algorithm [KP08]. For example, tinnitus dataset contains multiple instances that refer to one unique object (patient with

Table 4.3 Action rules generated from 2-element τ and δ [IR08]

τ	δ	sup	$conf$	$rule$
$(b_1 \wedge d_2) \Longrightarrow$	$(b_2 \wedge d_1)$	1	1	y
$(b_1 \wedge d_2) \Longrightarrow$	$(b_2 \wedge d_3)$	1	1	y
$(b_1 \wedge d_2) \Longrightarrow$	$(b_3 \wedge d_1)$	1	1	y
$(b_2 \wedge d_1) \Longrightarrow$	$(b_1 \wedge d_2)$	1	1	y
$(b_2 \wedge d_3) \Longrightarrow$	$(b_1 \wedge d_1)$	1	1	y
$(b_2 \wedge d_3) \Longrightarrow$	$(b_1 \wedge d_2)$	1	1	y
$(b_2 \wedge d_3) \Longrightarrow$	$(b_3 \wedge d_1)$	1	1	y
$(b_3 \wedge d_1) \Longrightarrow$	$(b_1 \wedge d_2)$	1	1	y
$(b_3 \wedge d_1) \Longrightarrow$	$(b_2 \wedge d_3)$	1	1	y
$(c_1 \wedge d_3) \Longrightarrow$	$(c_2 \wedge d_1)$	1	1	y

Table 4.4 Invalid transitions generated from 2-element τ and δ [IR08]

τ	δ	sup	$conf$	$rule$
$(b_1 \wedge d_1) \Longrightarrow$	$(b_2 \wedge d_3)$	1	0.33	n
$(c_2 \wedge d_1) \Longrightarrow$	$(c_1 \wedge d_3)$	1	0.25	n
$(a_1 \wedge d_1)$	$(a_1 \wedge d_1)$			
$(a_1 \wedge d_2)$	$(a_1 \wedge d_2)$			
$(a_1 \wedge d_3)$	$(a_1 \wedge d_3)$			
$(a_2 \wedge d_1)$	$(a_2 \wedge d_1)$			

multiple recordings of visits). The instances of data are also coupled with timestamps. For this reason, let assume that $I_S(x)$ denotes all instances of object x in an information system S. We should also define relation $\subseteq I_S(x) \times I_S(x)$ as: $((x_1, x_2) \in \subseteq)$ iff (x_2 occurred after x_1). Next, a temporal constraint for the algorithm should be defined: assuming that the only valid change of attribute value is the change that happens between two instances of the same object, where we limit the transition direction to occur from an earlier observation to a more recent one. For example, if we have two observations x_1 and x_2, where x_2 occurred after x_1, we will only consider change of state from x_1 to x_2. Next, we also define object-driven assumption, that is, assumption that a group of all instances for any unique object p is an independent subsystem by itself. Consequently, the action rules that we extract from the overall system are the result of aggregating action rules from all subsystems.

Table 4.5 3-Element τ and δ [IR08]

τ	δ
$(a_2 \wedge b_1 \wedge d_1)$	$(a_1 \wedge c_2 \wedge d_3)$
$(a_2 \wedge c_3 \wedge d_1)$	$(a_1 \wedge b_2 \wedge d_3)$
$(a_1 \wedge b_1 \wedge d_1)$	$(b_2 \wedge c_2 \wedge d_3)$
$(a_1 \wedge c_3 \wedge d_1)$	
$(b_1 \wedge c_3 \wedge d_1)$	

Table 4.6 Action rules generated from 3-element τ and δ [IR08]

τ	δ	sup	$conf$	$rule$
$(a_1 \wedge b_1 \wedge d_1) \implies$	$(a_1 \wedge b_2 \wedge d_3)$	1	1	y
$(a_1 \wedge c_3 \wedge d_1) \implies$	$(a_1 \wedge c_2 \wedge d_3)$	1	1	y
$(b_1 \wedge c_3 \wedge d_1) \implies$	$(b_2 \wedge c_2 \wedge d_3)$	1	1	y

Table 4.7 Invalid transitions generated from 3-element τ and δ [IR08]

τ	δ	sup	$conf$	$rule$
$(a_2 \wedge b_1 \wedge d_1) \implies$	$(a_1 \wedge b_2 \wedge d_3)$	1	0.50	n
$(a_2 \wedge c_3 \wedge d_1) \implies$	$(a_1 \wedge c_2 \wedge d_3)$	1	0.33	n

	τ	δ
Table 4.8 4-Element τ and δ and corresponding action rule [IR08]	$(a_2 \wedge b_1 \wedge c_3 \wedge d_1) \implies$	$(a_1 \wedge b_2 \wedge c_3 \wedge d_3)$

4.5 Meta Actions

Action rules are mined on the entire set of objects in S. Meta-actions, on the other hand, are chosen based on the action rules. They are formally defined as higher level concepts used to model a generalization of action rules in an information system [RW00]. They trigger actions that cause transitions in values of some flexible attributes in the information system. These changes, in turn, result in a change of decision attributes' values.

4.5.1 Definition

Definition 4.7 Let $M(S)$ be a set of meta-actions associated with an information system S. Let $a \in A$, $x \in X$, and $M \subset M(S)$. Applying the meta-actions in the set M on object x will result in $M(a(x)) = a(y)$, where object x is converted to object y by applying all meta-actions in M to x.

Example 4.3 Let $M(S)$, where $S = (X, A)$, be a set of meta-actions associated with an information system S. In addition let $T = \{v_{i,j} : j \in J_i, x_i \in X\}$ be the set of ordered transactions, patient visits, such that $v_{i,j} = [(x_i, A(x_i)_j)]$, where $A(x_i)_j$ is a set of attribute values $\{a(x_i) : a \in A\}$ of the object x_i for the visit represented uniquely by the visit identifier j. Each visit represents the current state of the object (patient) and current diagnosis. For each patient's two consecutive visits $(v_{i,j}, v_{i,j+1})$, where meta-actions were applied at visit j, it is possible to extract an *action set*. In this example, an *action set* is understood as an expression that defines a change of state for a distinct attribute that takes several values (multivalued attribute) at any object state. For example $\{a_1, a_2, a_3\} \rightarrow \{a_1, a_4\}$ is an action set that defines a change of values for attribute $a \in A$ from the set $\{a_1, a_2, a_3\}$ to $\{a_1, a_4\}$, where $\{a_1, a_2, a_3, a_4\} \subseteq V_a$ [TRSW14].

These action sets resulting from the application of meta-actions represent the actionable knowledge needed by practitioners. However, not every patient reacts in the same way to the same meta-actions, because each of them may have different preconditions. In other words, some patients might be partially affected by the meta actions and might have other side-effects. There emerges a need to introduce personalization on meta actions when executing action rules. The problem of personalized meta-actions is a fairly new topic that creates room for new improvements. There has been very minor work on the personalization of meta-actions so far [Wan14]. Action sets have to be additionally mined for the historical patterns. To evaluate these action set patterns some frequency measure for all patients has to be used (for example support or confidence). There is a room for improvements in personalized meta action mining, as well. In healthcare for instance, meta actions representing patient's treatments, could be mined from doctor's prescription. In addition to action rule mining in healthcare, meta actions present an interesting area for personalized treatments mining and cure mining.

4.5.2   Discovery Methods

As being the actual solutions to trigger action rules and ultimately improve recovery of tinnitus patients, meta actions discovery is important role for the purpose of building recommender system for tinnitus. However, while there have been designed many strategies for action rules discovery and they are quite mature, mining for meta-actions still is opened to further developments and not many methods are known. One of the very recent method, based on text mining and sentiment analysis, is presented in [KDJR14] for the application of increasing customer satisfaction (so called "Net Promoter Score") for heavy equipment repair companies.

One approach for tinnitus treatment problem would be to assume that meta actions are already known (for example prescribing a particular sound generator as method of treatment) and concentrate on selecting those that led to desired effect, the similar way as in the [TRSW14]. Also, it is possible to perform text mining on textual attributes describing method of treatment for visits in detail (if available), in order to discover effective meta actions, similar way as applied in [KDJR14] for the exploration of textual opinions of clients on a company given in a form.

4.6   Advanced Clustering Techniques

Advanced clustering methods can be used in medical dataset with visits to group patients according to similar visits' frequencies (similar visits patterns). The goal would be, similar as in case of meta actions, further enhancement for treatment personalization (assuming that patients with similar visit frequencies are comparable in terms of improvement tracking). The approach assumes that patients should be clustered in such a way that the visiting history of each patient is discretized into durations, anchored from its initial visit date in terms of weeks, and serving as a seed for grouping.

Visit Distance

Let define a visit distance, as a time difference between initial visit and a current visit. For example, a patient p who visited a doctor on July 8th, 2009, August 14th, 2009, and October 7th, 2009, is denoted, in terms of visit distance, as in Table 4.9.

Table 4.9 An example of calculating visit duration

Visit ID	Duration(weeks)
1	6
2	14

The corresponding vector representation will have the form $v_p = [6, 14]$. It means that patient p visited the doctor five full weeks after his first visit and his last visit happened 13 weeks after his first visit (or 7 weeks after his second visit). In other words, patient p visited the doctor in the 6th week and 14th week counting in relation to his initial visit.

Distance Between Patients

Let us assume that patient p visits distances are denoted by a vector $v_p = [v_1, v_2, \ldots, v_n]$, and patient q visits—by a vector $v_q = [w_1, w_2, \ldots, w_m]$. If $n < m$, then the distance $\rho(p, q)$ between p, q and the distance $\rho(q, p)$ between q, p is defined as [ZRJT10]:

$$\rho(q, p) = \rho(p, q) = \frac{\sum_i^n |v_i - w_{J(i)}|}{n} \tag{4.1}$$

where $[w_{J(1)}, w_{J(2)}, \ldots, w_{J(n)}]$ is a subsequence of $[w_1, w_2, \ldots, w_m]$ such that $\sum_i^n |v_i - w_{J(i)}|$ is minimal for all n-element subsequences of $[w_1, w_2, \ldots, w_m]$. $|v_i - w_{J(i)}|$ means absolute value of $[v_i - w_{J(i)}]$.

For example, if patient p has 6 visits and patient q has 5 visits with frequencies denoted correspondingly by vectors: $v_p = [5, 8, 12, 20, 26]$, and $v_q = [7, 11, 13, 21]$, and we want to compare p with q, each of the four distances of q should be matched with a closest visit of p and their difference should be averaged. In the given example, we match $w_1 = 7$ with $v_1 = 5$ (difference = 2), $w_2 = 11$ with $v_2 = 8$ (difference = 3), $w_3 = 13$ with $v_3 = 12$ (difference = 1), and $w_4 = 21$ with $v_4 = 20$ (difference = 1). The average difference is then calculated as: $\frac{2+3+1+1}{4} = \frac{7}{4}$, that is distance $\rho(q, p)$ is about 2.

Tolerance Classes and Threshold

It can be checked that $\rho(q, p)$ is a tolerance relation. *Threshold* can be applied to filter out patient records with large distance values to form a tolerance class, where all group members have similar visiting patterns [ZRJT10].

For instance, let us assume that we have 8 patients $p_1, p_2, p_3, \ldots, p_8$ with doctor's visits assigned to them which are represented by following vectors:

$v_{p_1} = [3, 8, 12, 20]$, $v_{p_2} = [4, 7]$, $v_{p_3} = [5, 12, 21, 30]$, $v_{p_4} = [7, 21, 29]$, $v_{p_5} = [12, 22]$, $v_{p_6} = [13, 19, 29]$, $v_{p_7} = [2, 13, 19, 31, 38]$, $v_{p_8} = [7, 12, 20]$.

The threshold value $\rho = 1$ is set up as a minimal distance between vectors representing patients.

The following tolerance classes containing more than one element will be constructed:

$TC_{\rho=1}(v_{p_2}) = [v_{p_1}, v_{p_2}]$, $TC_{\rho=1}(v_{p_4}) = [v_{p_4}, v_{p_3}]$, $TC_{\rho=1}(v_{p_5}) = [v_{p_5}, v_{p_1}, v_{p_3}, v_{p_8}]$, $TC_{\rho=1}(v_{p_6}) = [v_{p_6}, v_{p_7}]$, $TC_{\rho=1}(v_{p_6}) = [v_{p_6}, v_{p_1}]$.

We say that $TC_{\rho=1}(v_{p_2})$ is generated by p_2, and analogously, $TC_{\rho=1}(v_{p_4})$ is generated by p_4.

The ultimate goal of building tolerance classes, by a procedure presented above, is to identify groups of patients, for which temporally related features of tinnitus indicators, can be constructed. Threshold value can be manipulated, in order to change the size of classes (if threshold value is increased, the tolerance classes get larger). The size of tolerance classes should not be too small so that to still be able to retrieve useful information through the knowledge extraction process. On the other hand, the larger the tolerance classes, the less accurate information in temporally related features.

Dataset Clusters

The dataset associated with a tolerance class which is generated by patient p contains records describing patients who visited the doctor at similar weeks as the patient p. Data referring only to these visits should be stored as tuples representing all patients in this tolerance class. For example, if patient p generates a tolerance class $TC_{\rho=1}(v_{p_2})$, where $v_{p_2} = [4, 7]$, and another patient p_1 has a vector representation $v_{p_1} = [3, 8, 12, 20]$ of their doctor's visits, then p_1 has a vector representation $[3, 8]$ relative to $TC_{\rho=1}(v_{p_2})$. Thus, all patients associated with the same tolerance class have the same number of doctor's visits and all these visits occurred approximately at the same time (in relation to the start of treatment).

The goal of such approach is to construct a collection of databases D_p, where p is a patient and D_p corresponds to $TC_{\rho=1}(v_{p_2})$, for the purpose of knowledge discovery (classifier construction and rules extraction).

Algorithmic Approach for Clustering

Another approach is to represent each patient as a vector of distances between consecutive visits. In the example above $v_p = [5, 8 - 5, 12 - 8, 20 - 12, 26 - 20] = [5, 3, 4, 8, 6]$, and $v_q = [7, 11 - 7, 13 - 11, 21 - 13] = [7, 4, 2, 8]$. Instead of matching visits, we can translate the problem to the problem of finding optimal "cut points" so that to minimize distance between p and q. For example, we might choose following cut points: $v_p = [5|3|4|8|6]$ and $v_q = [7|4|2|8]$. The number of cut point for v_p is 4, and for v_q − 3. The corresponding distance is calculated as: $\frac{|(7)-(5)|+|(4)-(3)|+|(2)-(4)|+|(8)-(8)|}{4} = \frac{2+1+2+0}{4} = \frac{5}{4}$. Or we might choose another combination of cut points: $v_p = [5, 3|4|8|6]$ and $v_q = [7|4|2, 8)]$. This time we cut v_p with 3 points, and v_q with 2. Then the corresponding distance is calculated as: $\frac{|(5+3)-(7)|+|(4)-(4)|+|(8)-(2+8)|}{4} = \frac{1+0+2}{4} = \frac{3}{4}$. As we can see, we might choose different number of cuts.

The problem of "finding cuts" complicates, when an assumption is taken, that number of cuts can be any positive integer k, such that $k < n$, where n is a length of visit distance vector for a patient p, with a lower number of visits ($n < m$). Then, for each such k, each combination of k cut points in v_p with each combination of l cut points in v_q must be taken to calculate $\rho(q, p)$, where l creates a subsequence of a vector v_q of the length the same as subsequence of a vector v_p, created by k cut points creates a in v_p.

Procedure for Creating Dataset Clusters with Given Threshold

```
CREATE_CLUSTERS(number threshold, ARRAY all_patients)
 clusters_set [ARRAY][ARRAY]
 for each patient p in Patients[ARRAY]:
   #for each number of possible cut points in V_p
   for k = 1  to len(V_p -1):
     for all possible subsequences in V_p with k
      cut points
       #create a new cluster
       create D_p_c[ARRAY]
       #where p is an identifier of a patient p
       #and c - of combination
       add tuple(V_p_c) to D_p_c[ARRAY]
       for each patient q in Patients[ARRAY]:
         if len(V_q) >= len(V_p_c)
             if MINIMAL_DISTANCE(V_p_c,V_q)
             < threshold
             add tuple(V_q) to D_p_c[ARRAY]
       add D_p_c[ARRAY] to clusters_set
```

Procedure Finding Minimal Distance Between Two Distance Vectors

```
MINIMAL_DISTANCE(vector V_p_c, vector V_q)
 set minDist = 9999
 find l - nr of cut points in V_q
 #such that len(V_q_l) = len(V_p_c)
 for all possible subsequences in V_q with l cut point
    choose next V_q_c subsequence
    calculate distance between V_q_c ,V_p_c
        if dist(V_q_c ,V_p_c) < minDist
            minDist = dist(V_q_c, V_p_c)
            #save tuple with associated subsequence
            set tuple(V_q) = tuple(V_q_c)
   return minDist
```

4.7 Conclusion

In this chapter, a theoretical background for knowledge discovery approach to build recommender system, including concepts of action rules, meta actions was presented. Also, recent strategies in action rule discovery were investigated, as well as challenges associated with the novelty of meta actions applications. Examples on application of these concepts and strategies to the domain of tinnitus diagnosis and treatment were given. Approach was proposed on how to adjust temporal medical datasets to the rule extraction algorithms, including techniques of patient clustering. We would like to point out that a number points out, a number and time of visits as factors should have some impact on treatment outcome, but it should not be decisive factor. As a rule of thumb, doctor needs at least 3 visits to confirm/contradict the prediction. As medical experience shows, not too much attention should be paid to this measure, while other parameters could be dominant. "Distance between patients" is a useful measure in the normal practice where time of visits is very varied. In clinical trials the distance would be zero. The problem is that in normal clinic there is large variability of the number of visit. Typically, the last visits are more important and they will be ignored for patients with large number of visits. As for "tolerance classes" it is possible to expect continuum of distances without clear subgrouping—so without clear thresholds.

    In summary the pattern of visits should not be the only factor considered. This factor should have Yes/No type of discrimination, with likelihood of success more probably for number of visit larger then (e.g. 3). It does not have impact on categorization of patients, while it is possible to predict some nonlinear relation with severity of tinnitus and presence of DST.

    This chapter closes theoretical part of this book.

Chapter 5
RECTIN System Design

Abstract RECTIN system (shortcut for RECommender for TINnitus) is a prototyping method proposed within this work to verify the hypothesis of possibility to apply information technology in supporting physicians, dealing with tinnitus patients, in the diagnosis and treatment. This chapter describes major steps in the system design: analysis with main use cases for the system, deployment architecture, with detailed description of each component and implementation project, including transactional database and application. Also, knowledge engineering approach is presented, along with detailed description of raw dataset of tinnitus patients and visits, which was made available to the authors. This section also introduces approach taken to data preprocessing so that to make it useful for creating a knowledge base, on which data mining can be performed.

5.1 System Analysis

Processes in medical facility supported with RECTIN system include (Fig. 5.1):

- Collecting data about patients and their visits at medical facility. Data collected includes demographic information, medical information (on pharmaceuticals taken and audiological measurements) and forms.
- Storing the data in the central database of medical facility.
- Performing characterization of tinnitus based on data collected from a patient at a visit and prediction models built on historical data.
- Advising in treatment actions with the use of rule engine facility.

The basic use case for RECTIN usage is a patient's visit at medical facility, where a physician firstly conducts an interview with a patient and enters data about his/her demographics, medical condition, tinnitus induction (at initial visit), or comments and outcomes, as well as different indicators' measurements for consecutive visits. Patients should, on the other hand, fill out electronic forms (initial/follow-up

© Springer International Publishing AG 2017
K.A. Tarnowska et al., *Decision Support System for Diagnosis and Treatment of Hearing Disorders*, Studies in Computational Intelligence 685,
DOI 10.1007/978-3-319-51463-5_5

Fig. 5.1 Use cases for
RECTIN system

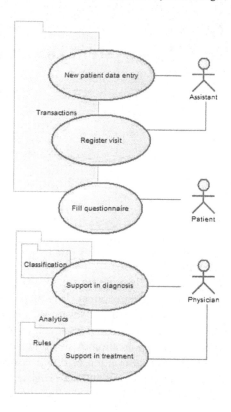

forms and Newman form), based on paper version as in Appendix A, B and C. However, when confronted with our medical practice, these forms are actually serving as a help to perform structural interviews and patients should not be doing them. Therefore, the modification to the system can be that physician performing interview fills out the electronic forms. The new data, entered both by a physician/medical facility assistant and by a patient/physician through electronic form, is inserted into the central database server. Then the classification module and action rules module should match and generate, correspondingly, diagnostic and treatment recommendation, based on the new data from patient and previously constructed models/inserted rules. The recommendation is shown to a physician who decides on the final diagnosis and treatment, which ultimately applies to the patient. The system will all the time modify itself on the base of new data.

5.2 System Architecture

Figure 5.2 depicts a high-level architecture and basic data flow for RECTIN system deployed within the medical facility treating tinnitus patients.

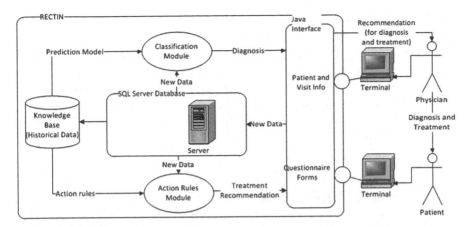

Fig. 5.2 Architecture and data flow in deployment diagram of RECTIN

The system is assumed to be built as a window application storing data in a database server. Java interface should be enabled on end terminals. Central database would allow for concurrent transactions for many users, as it is assumed that both physicians and patients filling out the forms can update the data simultaneously. Central database should therefore provide data integrity and security.

5.2.1 Knowledge Base

Knowledge module consists of historical data of patients and their visits collected in medical facility in Atlanta in years 1999–2005. It is separated from the transactional database, as it is stored in structures convenient for data analysis, data mining and machine learning. The raw data needs cleaning and transformation before it could be used for building prediction models or rule extraction. It is assumed that knowledge base should be also updated with the new data, and "relearn" its models (automatic data acquisition functionality).

5.2.2 Classification Module

Classification module is supposed to perform diagnosis prediction (categorization) for a new patient, based on previously learned model. Before implementing particular classifier, tests should be conducted in order to compare and choose the best classification model, in terms of accuracy and F-score, on the given dataset. The module's main functionality is to suggest category of tinnitus, to which a patient should be assigned, in an automatic and reliable way and thus support physician's opinion.

5.2.3   Action Rules Module

Action rules module consists of rules and should implement rules engine (for automatic inference). It is assumed that rules can be hard-coded and evoked based on matching with the new data. Rules extraction should be tested in experiments, so that to obtain rules with the best support and confidence. The aim is to present treatment actions to the system user, which should lead to patient's improvement, given his current medical condition.

5.3   Knowledge Engineering

The given dataset on tinnitus patients and their visits has to be preprocessed, transformed and cleaned, before it can be useful for data mining and machine learning purposes. The original dataset is organized into 11 separate Access-format tables. The dataset presents several challenges. Firstly, the original data is not in a relational form. It means that data about a particular visit, that resides in different tables, is not related with foreign keys. Furthermore, data is in many cases inconsistent (lacking integrity) along different tables and there are numerous errors in visits' dates, visits numbering etc. (therefore it is also impossible to create foreign keys without data loss and errors). It apparently resulted from error-prone manual data entering (entering data from paper forms, which, handwritten, could have been not clearly visible to the person entering the data). For example, tuples with the same patient identifier and visit number have different *Date* values in different tables (by means of days, months and even years)—which proved to be quite problematic while merging the data. It required manual checking and fixing. Taking into account about 3000 tuples with visits, this process turned out to be time-consuming and arduous. However, the correctness and thus accuracy of the data had to be assured, before any knowledge could be extracted from the dataset, as inaccurate data would yield consequently unreliable knowledge and analytical conclusions.

In order to make data suitable for data mining, one matrix or one big table needs to be created, by means of merging data residing in 11 separate tables (Fig. 5.3 shows 10 of them, missing *Visits* table). The aim is to retain the informational content (avoid information loss while merging tuples with missing values). The preprocessing task proved to be quite cumbersome and problematic, mainly on the grounds presented in the paragraph above.

The Fig. 5.3 presents original table structure that groups data into areas, described in the following subsection.

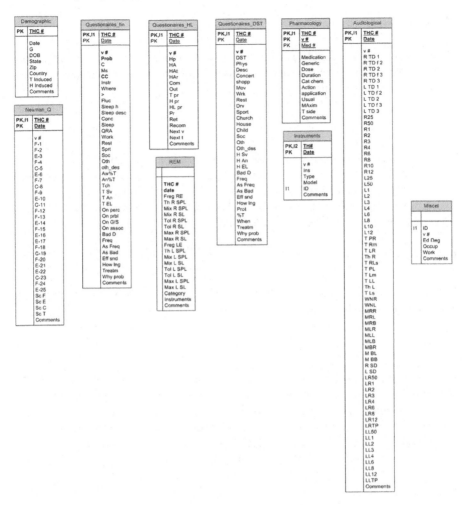

Fig. 5.3 Tinnitus patients and visits dataset structure in original format [Tho11]

5.3.1 Raw Data

Demographics

Demographics information, such as address data, age, gender, etc. These are mostly nominal data, but the table contains columns with textual descriptions as well (of special interest would be those describing tinnitus onset). It is also worth mentioning that the raw data had already been anonymized, that is, personal identifiable information (such as name, surname, insurance number) had already been removed before leaving the medical facility.

Miscellaneous

Miscellaneous table—could be understood as complementary to demographics, containing information about patient's occupation, work status and some textual information entered at discretion.

Pharmacology

Contains information about particular medications taken by a patient when the treatment on tinnitus started. Information on medications, their generic names, prescribed doses and the underlying medical condition was mostly collected at initial visit. Therefore, information in this table can be helpful in discovering knowledge on how additional, independent afflictions can influence tinnitus categorization.

Instruments

Instruments table—contains details about instruments used in tinnitus treatment along with the details as for the type, model, etc.

Audiological

Audiological information contains all the medical measurements carried out by the doctor either at diagnosis at initial visit or at further visits when controlling the medical condition of the patient. The details on the meaning of each measurement is outside of scope of this work, because it is based on technical knowledge in medicine and audiology. The values are numerical, but can be grouped or discretized as these columns contain limited number of distinct values.

NewmanQ

NewmanQ table makes an important inventory of initial tinnitus severity and its change during treatment allowing for monitoring treatment progress (based on Tinnitus Handicap Inventory form in Appendix C). The shortcuts in columns' names containing a letter and a number designate a particular question related to the patient's subjective opinion on the tinnitus impact on one of the three important areas of their life: emotional (E), functional (F) and catastrophical (C). Basically, the column names reflect the form structure (see Appendix C). Each answer is evaluated with numerical value interpreted as "no", "sometimes" or "yes". Summary points for each area are reflected in $Sc\ F$, $Sc\ E$, $Sc\ C$ columns, and in $Sc\ T$ as a total score of all of them. According to our medical expertise, subscales are not useful and that only total score should be used. This summary value holds very important information about subjective tinnitus severity level (described in Appendix C). Changes in $Sc\ T$ can be considered patient's tinnitus improvement or deterioration, so can be used for tracking the treatment actions' effectiveness. It also somehow correlates with the category of tinnitus severity that is assigned by a doctor (it allows to classify patients into Category 0, for all other categories can be the same). This measure is of key importance, as the aim of the decision support system built within this work, is to find actions (and action rules) in medical treatment that lead to decrease in total score value.

Questionnaire tin, Questionnaire HL, Questionnaire DST

These tables can be interpreted analogously as the NewmanQ table—they reflect the structure of the particular form—in this case "Tinnitus initial interview form" (see Appendix A) or "Tinnitus follow-up interview form" (see Appendix B), depending whether the visit was initial or subsequent. The interview form, both initial and follow-up, is basically divided into three sections: tinnitus, sound tolerance and hearing problem, which are filled, accordingly, whether a patient is affected by the problem. These three sections of the form are reflected in the corresponding three tables in the dataset. When paper versions of the forms (Appendices A and B) are compared to the tables' structures in Fig. 5.3, it becomes more apparent. The answers on the forms' questions are Likert scale, for example between 0 and 10. But textual comments written on the sheets are also entered into the database and provide additional information. These tables contain the largest number of errors. Although, so far, paper forms' content has been entered manually into the database, the ultimate solution would be electronic forms that could automatically update information in the central database, avoiding the problem of human typing errors and human handwriting recognition errors. The alternative that could help in entering accurate data would be to use hand-written characters recognition software, which is, nevertheless, not that reliable as data entered electronically.

Visits

Visits table constitutes a basic inventory of visits and their outcomes. It is important source of the data in preprocessing as often serves as the most reliable source of temporal data (dates) and accurate visit enumeration.

REM

REM table stores sound level as set by a patient at a given visit, representing important treatment actions. Each setting parameter is very important and has impact on treatment outcome.

5.3.2   Data Preprocessing

The approach taken to merge the data from different tables into one data table included importing Access-format data to the Microsoft Server database management system and performing SQL FULL OUTER JOIN operations on consecutive tables. Example of the join operation on the tables is shown on the listing below.

Listing 5.1   Sample SQL JOIN operation on separate data.

```
1   SELECT  COALESCE(THC_a#,  TH#)  AS  THC#,  COALESCE(v_a#,  vi#)  AS  v#,
2                   COALESCE(A.Date_a,  Date_i)  AS  Date,  *
3   INTO  dbo.AudInstT
4   FROM    Tinnitus.dbo.Audiological  as  A  FULL  OUTER  JOIN
5                          Tinnitus.dbo.Instruments  as  I
6   ON  A.THC_a#  =  I.TH#  AND  A.v_a#  =  I.vi#
```

By using OUTER JOIN a new database was created without information loss (data was retained regardless whether it had corresponding values in another table). Each JOIN operation had to be considered separately and different join attributes were chosen to provide the best accuracy of the joint tuples (for example, one time, it was only visit ID, another time visit ID along with the visit date). After such operations of creating bigger tables, additional manual checks were performed to assure correctness of the newly created tuples. In order to reduce the number of "empty" visits, some simplifying assumptions were made. For example, audiological measurements and forms performed in just one day difference were merged into one tuple (as both represent evaluation, not treatment actions). Also, most REM data contained dates that seemed to be entered into the system with one-day delay in relation to the visits' dates (frequently initial visit lasted two days), therefore, was treated as those visits' attribute, rather than new visit tuple, which would be very sparse. On some conflicting or missing data, common reasoning, as well as more detailed analysis of the particular patient case and their visits, was applied. To be able to perform more complicated merging of data, PLSQL procedures were developed and applied rather than doing manual check.

As a final result, one big table was created with redundant data in columns (structure convenient for performing analytics). Each tuple represents a patient's visit and is characterized by the patient's data (which therefore repeats for each visit) and visit-specific data, such as treatment performed at a particular visit (counseling, instrumentation, instrument fitting), medical measurements and forms completed either at that visit or shortly before or after the visit. As practically each of the 11 merged tables contained textual comment column (see Fig. 5.3), the single resulting table had to be simplified, firstly, by excluding columns unsuitable for automatic classifiers. However, it is assumed to perform some basic feature extraction from text attributes before initial experiments on data mining.

Analyzing such a complex dataset with so many attributes is vital to further development and enhancement of RECTIN system. The structure where data should be stored ultimately, has to be redesigned, so that to ensure efficiency of transactional operation in RECTIN (inserting, retrieving data, minimizing storage).

5.4 Summary

This chapter presented RECTIN system analysis, design and deployment plan, with most important associations and data flows between particular components and use cases for the system. Important step in developing a knowledge base for a rule-based recommender system is a knowledge engineering process, which includes data analysis and preprocessing. Raw data cleansing and transforming it into usable form proves to be a time-consuming and arduous task, which should be avoided by proper structuring data entry in future implementation of the method. Majority of data are ordinal (Likert scales—e.g. subjective ranking of tinnitus loudness, annoyance) and some are ratio, e.g., % of time of tinnitus awareness, % of time of tinnitus annoyance. All audiometric data are on ration scale. Although many attributes are nominal (and the numerical ones can be turned to nominal), text columns with potentially useful information also exist. There comes the need for text mining and feature extraction. Some automatic methods of text extraction can be applied, but in order to obtain possibly the most complete information, it rather requires to be checked and entered manually, which however proves to be a quite time-consuming task.

Providing an overview of initial steps in working with data, the chapter introduces us to the next one, which will present initial experiments on the prepared cleansed dataset.

Chapter 6
Experiment 1: Classifiers

Abstract Following the dataset preprocessing, the next step in implementing RECTIN is classification module development. The classification module will use a model built on historical patients' data, in order to support physicians in suggesting optimal treatment approach for new patients. Categorization is rather easy and relatively broad. However, a specific approach within each category varies. Before implementing this module, it is necessary to extract new, useful features and conduct experiments in order to obtain the most accurate classifier on the prepared dataset. It is assumed to reiterate the step of feature development in order to obtain the best combination of feature extraction/selection method and the prediction method. This involves the calibration and tuning of prediction methods, as well as comparing them and evaluating in terms of accuracy, F-score and confusion matrix.

6.1 Initial Feature Development

As the first goal of tinnitus data analysis is to find a reliable classifier for tinnitus characterization, it has to be determined which attributes would be most relevant in diagnosis decision-making process, as well as those that could form patterns, novel to a doctor himself. There are international norms classifying tinnitus patient to specific category. For example, a doctor may follow decision-making rules that relate forms output to a particular tinnitus category. However having hundreds of patients, it is very unlikely that he remembers each patients' additional affliction, such as diabetics or asthma, or medication taken, so that to apply this additional knowledge on patients' characteristics, to diagnosis decision for a new patient. Therefore, from machine learning point of view, it would be interesting to discover not only a good classifier that is based on obvious knowledge, but also decision rules that are hidden beyond large amounts of patients' data. This is why some additional features were extracted before performing initial experiments on the dataset.

© Springer International Publishing AG 2017

K.A. Tarnowska et al., *Decision Support System for Diagnosis and Treatment of Hearing Disorders*, Studies in Computational Intelligence 685, DOI 10.1007/978-3-319-51463-5_6

6.1.1 Tinnitus Background

Important question that is asked by a doctor at the initial visit is related to the background or main cause associated with an onset of tinnitus symptoms. This information was saved in the database in text columns, making it inappropriate for classification algorithms. Therefore, new binary attributes were developed based on the textual descriptions in *T Induced* and *H Induced* columns in the *Demographics* table. The binary attributes convey information whether patient's tinnitus was induced by a cause given by the attribute:

- *STI*—Stress Tinnitus Induced—whether tinnitus was induced by stressful situations in a patient's life. This category includes cases described as 'divorce', 'excessive work', 'moved into new house', 'stress over terrorist attacks', 'after graduation', etc.
- *NTI*—Noise Tinnitus Induced—whether tinnitus was induced by noise. This category includes patients described with, for example, 'noise exposure', 'military involvement, shooting practice', 'after playing in a band', 'shooting guns'.

Other binary attributes developed to indicate tinnitus/hyperacusis cause were related to specific medical conditions:

- *HLTI*—Hearing Loss Tinnitus Induced—covers patients who associated their tinnitus with hearing loss.
- *DETI*—Depression Tinnitus Induced—relates tinnitus symptoms to depression.
- *AATI*—Auto Accident Tinnitus Induced—whether tinnitus emerged as a result of auto accident, which involved head injuries.
- *OTI*—Operation Tinnitus Induced—patients after surgeries.
- *OMTI*—Other Medical—patients, whose tinnitus was related to medical conditions other than hearing loss, depression or operation—patients with acoustic neuroma, Lyme's disease, ear infections, obsessive compulsive disorder and others.

There were also patients described with more than one cause, for example, the patient described as 'was in the military' was given 'True' value in both *STI* and *NTI* columns. Tinnitus of a patient who experienced gunshot could be described as induced by all the conditions: stress, noise and medical condition (because of the injury resulted from the shot). Also, different medical conditions could be related to each other, for example a patient after auto accident could most probably have undergone a surgery. Unfortunately, there is about one third of patients' tuples whose tinnitus was not described at all in terms of its roots (value for *T induced* column was NULL). This is because idiopathic tinnitus is very common.

Another potentially interesting information that could be extracted from *T induced* column was whether tinnitus appeared suddenly or developed gradually over time. Unfortunately most cases were not described by these terms, so these are very sparse columns.

6.1.2 Temporal Features for Tinnitus Induction

Another information that could be useful for a doctor, for both treatment and diagnosis purposes, is patient's age. Having information about patient's date of birth, as well as date of the first visit, a column, informing what was the age of the patient when they started treatment, can be derived. After some data analysis, it was observed that some patients went to doctor immediately after tinnitus onset, while the others had been suffering from it for a long time before they came to doctor Jastreboff. However, according our medical knowledge, in case of TRT age is irrelevant, except when it is related to brain plasticity. Temporal information could be also extracted from *T induced* column (or *H induced*), which often contains data about what time ago or the date the tinnitus (or hyperacusis) appeared. This proved to be quite problematic for an automatic extraction, as some tuples were described as "ago", while the others were given the specific date. It took some time, therefore, to develop new attributes:

- *DTI*—Date Tinnitus Induced (from column *T induced*), and
- *DHI*—Date Hyperacusis Induced (from column *H induced*).

Each tuple for separate patients was checked for that information, manually calculated and entered into new columns. But, having this information it was possible to derive a number of new features: the age of a patient when tinnitus started, as well as the time elapse between tinnitus onset and initial visit to doctor. It can potentially lead to discovering the knowledge on an impact of patient's age at the start of the treatment, the age when tinnitus began, and time elapse from tinnitus symptoms' onset to treatment start, on the effectiveness of particular treatment methods in TRT (these are important points discussed in the literature, but results of our medical practice argue against them). For example, it may turn out, that elderly patients need different type of treatment protocol than the younger patient groups. It might also be true that the longer the tinnitus was not treated with TRT the smaller chances of success. These are just potential hypotheses, which nevertheless have to be proved with machine learning algorithms, and then with expert knowledge.

To summarize the work on temporal features development, following new columns were added to the original database:

- *DTI*—Date Tinnitus Induced—date column derived from text columns,
- *DHI*—Date Hyperacusis Induced—analogous to the above, but derived from *H induced* column—both these new attributes convey general information about when "the problem" started and both were developed manually,
- *AgeInd*—patient's age when the problem (tinnitus or hyperacusis) was induced—derived from *DOB* and *DTI/DHI* columns,
- *AgeBeg*—patient's age when they started TRT treatment (first visit to doctor Jastreboff) — derived from *DOB* and *Date* (of visit 0) columns,
- Numerical columns *DAgo*, *WAgo*, *MAgo*, *YAgo*—informing how many days, weeks, months, and years ago the problem started,
- Binary columns calculated on the basis of columns above: *Y30*, *Y20*, *Y10*, *Y5*, *Y3*, *Y1*, *M6*, *M3*, *M1*, *W2*, *W1*, *D1* informing to which group of time elapse, between

the tinnitus onset to treatment start, a patient belongs (Y—years, M—months, W—weeks, D—days, and numerical value). For example, having "True" value in $Y5$ column for the given patient, means that the problem was induced between 5 to 10 years before starting TRT treatment.

Presented approach for feature extraction provides just an example and outlook how potentially useful information can be extracted from textual columns and suggests directions for further work on the dataset. For example, similar work can be done on *Pharmacology* table, with regards to medications, a patient takes (can be developed into columns, instead of being column values), as well as accompanying afflictions and medical conditions. Also, it may be useful to determine numerical values of medicines' doses taken by a patient and time duration they were taken. It is important to have information related to brain function, e.g. Lyme disease, autism spectrum disorders. Still, most of such potentially interesting information is in textual form, making it useless for machine learning algorithms in the current form.

6.2 Preliminary Experiments

Experiments on classification were conducted with WEKA technology [BFH+14]. It offers a wide choice of prediction algorithms (and data mining algorithms in general), as well as friendly user interface and possibility to build a complete "knowledge flow", starting from reading the file with data, through feature selection, up to building a classification model, evaluating and visualizing the results. It also allows to use API (Java libraries containing the same classes that are available within the GUI), which can be helpful when incorporating the classifier model into a recommender system.

6.2.1 Assumptions

In the first experimental setup, it is assumed that each visit represents different object (and there is no temporal dependence between particular visits). In such transformed data representation, each patient's data is "multiplied" by number of visits and by number of medications they take. The decision attribute is C attribute—category of tinnitus assigned by a doctor. Example of experimental setup, in WEKA knowledge flow, is shown in Fig. 6.1.

The data is loaded from the prepared csv file, "CrossValidationFoldMaker" splits the data into test and training sets, which are inputs to chosen classifiers— RandomForest and J48 (tree-based algorithms). Constructed models are evaluated with cross-validation method (with 10 folds) and results are shown in either textual or visual form (tree graphs).

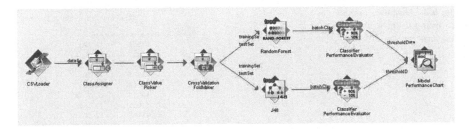

Fig. 6.1 Knowledge flow for comparing two tree classifiers' performance in WEKA

6.2.2 Feature Selection

The relevant attributes chosen for csv file included: audiological measurement, demographics, pharmacology, forms. The visit and patient identifiers are not relevant, as well as visit's date column. Moreover, all attributes that could be understood as the outcomes of the diagnosis decision, so all the actions regarding treatment methods (instruments, settings, etc.) were also omitted. Although they correlate with the patient's category, they would distort the prediction results, as should be considered rather results of diagnosis or action taken in response to it, than its premises and factors influencing patient's category. The columns with mostly (or only) NULL values were removed from the analysis as well.

After limiting the number of attributes in the csv file manually, the next step was to use automatic feature selector. WEKA contains feature selection algorithms that enable to rank attributes and choose a subset of them for the classification model construction. Experiment on the dataset with attribute evaluator set to "ChiSquaredAtributeEval" (based on chi-squared measure) and search method set to "Ranker" resulted in the attribute rank, as shown in Fig. 6.2 (only subset of best ranked is shown). It can be concluded that the most important features in determining patient's category are: their age (*DOB* attribute), as well time elapse since the problem started (attributes *DAgo*, *WAgo*, *MAgo*, *DTI*—Date Tinnitus induced, *DHI*—Date Hyperacusis Induced). It seems that age at which the problem started (attribute *AgeBeg*) also affects patient's category, although it does not make sense clinically—it may be linked via hearing loss which is correlated with age. Quite surprisingly place of residence (*Zip* attribute) seems to be relevant to diagnosis (according to our medical knowledge it does not make any sense so it may be just a result of data structure). Other factors observed to have an impact on patient's category include medications prescribed to the patient and corresponding generics taken, main problem (*P*)—(and according to medical knowledge it should be a dominant factor), occupation, then audiological measurements—and it makes sense in medical terms as hearing loss and LDLs are crucial factors for diagnosis, as subsequently the most relevant factors in diagnosis.

Fig. 6.2 Attributes ranked according to chi-squared measure

```
                                      Chi-squared Ranking Filter

                              Ranked attributes:
                              725.05001      45 LR4
                              712.70417      29 Th L
                              688.00398      44 LR3
                              683.38374      43 LR2
                              683.09068      42 LR1
                              672.58042      23 T LR
                              670.57001      47 LR8
                              667.46635      52 LL3
                              618.93623      24 Th R
                              617.06273      51 LL2
                              606.21401      53 LL4
                              603.4837       50 LL1
                              589.86863      55 LL8
                              585.03241      54 LL6
                              581.71272      46 LR6
                              573.40413      49 LL50
                              572.54551      28 T LL
                              553.86731      48 LR12
                              534.10423      41 LR50
                              527.04316     116 P
                              493.95612      86 Prob
                              480.98386      56 LL12
                              474.4102       31 WNR
                              455.47575      32 WNL
                              410.45686       4 R2
                              393.19923      37 MLL
                              387.73904      33 MRR
```

6.2.3   Results

The basic experiment in WEKA on 6991 object instances described by 161 attributes (without feature selection) with J48 tree classifier brought cross-validated results (with 10 folds) with 88.27% correctly classified instances. Best precision was observed for class "4" and "0" (0.914 and 0.905 correspondingly) and the best recall for class "1" (0.937). Consequently, the best F-measure was observed for this class (0.911). Observation of built pruned decision tree model leads to conclusion that classification rules are based on age of patient, age when tinnitus was induced and audiological measures, but also on medications. From medical point of view this is an interesting outcome, while in clinical practice age and zip code are not considered as being significant; audiology—yes; medications—not really. However, there is some data showing difference in prevalence of tinnitus depending on localization within the USA. This may potentially explain correlation with zip code.

Next experiment was conducted with random forest classifier (of 100 trees each considering 8 random features), which proved to outperform J48 in terms of accuracy—89.17% correct predictions. ROC curve, being a result from an experiment depicted on diagram in Fig. 6.1, is shown in Fig. 6.3.

It compares False Positive Rate (X axis) to True Positive Rate (Y axis) between two classifiers: Random Tree and J48 tree, for the chosen category — "2".

Test on multilayer neural network classification model turned out to be too computational intensive for the given dataset, ended up in "out of memory" error. Taking

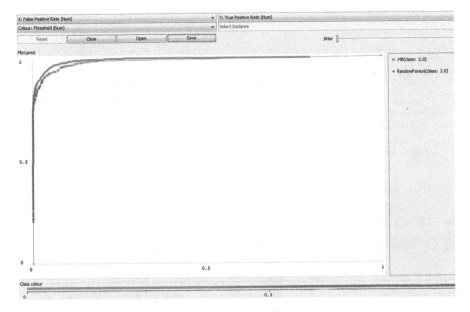

Fig. 6.3 ROC curve comparing classifiers based on J48 and Random Forest

into account cross-validation testing mode it would also took much more time to obtain results.

Decision table classifier performed with about 85% accuracy. Feature set considered in the model included: physical discomfort felt by a patient, tinnitus effect on work, patient's main problem (T/H/L), date of birth, patient's occupation and work status. Naive Bayes classifier performed worse than other classifiers, with 75.8% correctly classified instances.

Choosing discretization option in data preprocessing did not affect results significantly (mainly because most of attributes were already recognized as nominal).

Feature selection based on chi-squared measure slightly improved accuracy, but up to some number of attributes. Further limitation of attributes worsened accuracy. Cross correlations of the different attributes were not taken into account in this experimental setup. The details for different classifier (on experiment setup as shown in Fig. 6.4) are shown in Table 6.1.

Naive Bayes classifier brought the best accuracy with attribute reduction to about 20. Tree- and rule-based classifiers performed best when number of attributes was reduced by about half.

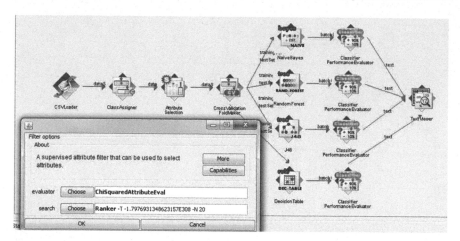

Fig. 6.4 Knowledge flow for classifier comparison with different feature selection settings

Table 6.1 Summary of experiments on feature selection/prediction method

Feature selection	J48 %	Random forest %	Decision table %	Naive Bayes %
No filter (161)	88.37	89.3	85.03	75.8
120	88.29		84.95	75.54
100	88.43	89.14	84.95	75.24
80	88.47	89.19	84.93	75.21
60	88.2	88.94	84.02	75.68
20	87.9	87.1	84.92	81.52

6.2.4 Discussion

The results obtained with the first experiments were quite optimistic, although it cannot be determined, whether good results come from dataset structure, which contains many repetitive instances for one patient (repeated with each visit and medication). It might be that in cross-validation testing, similar tuples were used for training and testing. In order to prove classifier validity, test set with new data would have to be delivered. However, WEKA options allow to test on data with exactly the same structure as training data. It requires not only the same attribute contents, but also exactly the same number of labels, as well the same order of labels for each nominal attribute. Therefore, attempts to manually split data set into separate (in terms of patients) train and test set proved to be too cumbersome (taking into account large number of attributes). Classifiers' reliability cannot be determined without new data, whose category prediction could be compared with an expert diagnosis. Therefore, further work on data preprocessing must be carried out (so that objects represent patients, not visits). The initial experiment helped to gain some outlook on feature selection and classification methodology choice and combination. Medical expertise confirms that if the aim is classification then only data from the first visit should be used. The category of the patient can change during the treatment, e.g., patients with tinnitus and hyperacusis (Category 3) can have hyperacusis removed and become Category 1 patients, then when severity of tinnitus decreases, become Category 0. In clinical practice medications are not affecting classification, while some medications, specifically benzodiazepines, have impact on treatment outcome.

6.3 Second Experimental Setup

Following conclusions from initial experiments and addressing questionable assumptions related to obtained classification results (as described in Discussion subsection of the previous section), further experiments were conducted, in order to verify classification results.

First and foremost problem associated with the previous experiments was related to dataset structure, on which prediction model was built. Each patient's data was repeated not only for every visit but also for every medication they take. In other words, a tuple with all the same, but different pharmacology attributes was considered different object. As a result, about 7000 were created out of about 500 distinct patients, and out of about 3000 distinct visits. This could have led to results' distortion, as testing method was based on cross-validation, where training and test sets were constructed in consecutive folds from the given dataset with many repetitive data. It means that it was highly probable that similar tuples were used both for training and for testing, which obviously overestimates accuracy (and medical expertise confirms that).

6.3.1 *Pharmacology Data Analysis*

In order to address problems with dataset, mentioned in the previous paragraph, dataset structure had to be changed. This will be particularly useful for the further analysis of treatment outcome.

First step in revising data structure was analyzing *Pharmacology* table, in terms of functional dependencies between particular columns. As depicted in Fig. 6.5, there are a number of potentially interesting columns to include for prediction model

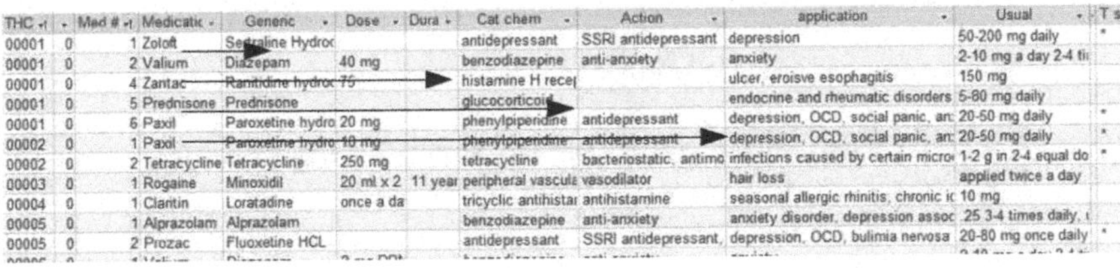

THC		Med #	Medicatic	Generic	Dose	Dura	Cat chem	Action	application	Usual	T side
00001	0	1	Zoloft	Sertraline Hydroc			antidepressant	SSRI antidepressant	depression	50-200 mg daily	*
00001	0	2	Valium	Diazepam	40 mg		benzodiazepine	anti-anxiety	anxiety	2-10 mg a day 2-4 ti	
00001	0	4	Zantac	Ranitidine hydroc	75		histamine H rece		ulcer, eroisve esophagitis	150 mg	
00001	0	5	Prednisone	Prednisone			glucocorticoid		endocrine and rheumatic disorders	5-80 mg daily	
00001	0	6	Paxil	Paroxetine hydro	20 mg		phenylpiperidine	antidepressant	depression, OCD, social panic, an	20-50 mg daily	*
00002	0	1	Paxil	Paroxetine hydro	10 mg		phenylpiperidine	antidepressant	depression, OCD, social panic, an	20-50 mg daily	*
00002	0	2	Tetracycline	Tetracycline	250 mg		tetracycline	bacteriostatic, antimo	infections caused by certain micro	1-2 g in 2-4 equal do	*
00003	0	1	Rogaine	Minoxidil	20 ml x 2	11 year	peripheral vascula	vasodilator	hair loss	applied twice a day	
00004	0	1	Claritin	Loratadine	once a da		tricyclic antihistar	antihistamine	seasonal allergic rhinitis, chronic ic	10 mg	
00005	0	1	Alprazolam	Alprazolam			benzodiazepine	anti-anxiety	anxiety disorder, depression assoc	.25 3-4 times daily,	
00005	0	2	Prozac	Fluoxetine HCL			antidepressant	SSRI antidepressant,	depression, OCD, bulimia nervosa	20-80 mg once daily	*

Fig. 6.5 Functional dependency analysis of Pharmacology table

construction. However, after closer insight, it seems that information in particular columns is functionally dependent (the table is not in the third normal form). The most important column is *Medication*, which then determines values in the *Generic* column, *Chemical category* column and *Action/Application* columns. Therefore, following functional dependencies can be established: "Medication → Generic", "Medication → Cat chem", "Medication → Action", "Medication → Application", "Medication → Usual" (see arrows in Fig. 6.5). *Action* and *Application* columns contain similar informational content, the latter being more descriptive. The only information that relates patient to medication is given by *Dose* and *Duration* columns (they contain quantitative description and temporal information of medication taken). *T side* column informs whether tinnitus developed as a side-effect of the medication uptake.

6.3.2 Pivotal Features Development

As analysis in the previous subsections shows, it is not necessary to develop all pharmacology's column values into new features, as patient's tuples with the same medication would be described by means of the same set of *Generic/Chemical/Action* attribute values.

Instead of maintaining a list of medications for each patient, they were altered into pivotal features (concept of pivoting the input data on a column value is depicted in Fig. 6.6).

By pivoting the data values on the medication column, the resulting set will contain a single row per patient. This single row lists all the medication taken by a patient, with the medication names shown as column names, and a binary value (True/False) for the columns. Also, *Dose* value could be stored, but it would be far more selective than simple binary values. Because not every patient takes every medication, the resulting matrix is very sparse.

Patient	Med#	Medication	Application
1	1	Zantac	ulcer
1	2	Valium	anxiety
1	3	Paxil	depression,OCD
2	1	Paxil	depression, anxiety

Pivotal form

Patient	Zantac	Valium	Paxil	Ulcer	Anxiety	Depression	OCD
1	1	1	1	1	1	1	1
2	0	0	1	0	1	1	0

Fig. 6.6 Illustration of pivoting idea applied on pharmacology attributes

Pivot transformation was deployed with PL/SQL procedures. Each distinct value in *Medication* column of *Pharmacology* table was developed into additional column. Bit values in the column indicate, for each patient-visit tuple, whether the medication denoted by a column name was taken (see Fig. 6.6). As a result, 311 additional features were developed, each for distinct medication. Alternatively, *Cat chem* could be used for the purpose of pivotal feature development, as it denotes more general chemical category of medications (there are 175 distinct chemical categories for 800 tuples in the *Pharmacology* table).

Similar approach was taken to *Application* column in *Pharmacology* table. Values in this column describe patients' medical problems that are associated with the taken medications. Thus, the column can also serve as a source of information about patient's additional diseases and afflictions, which should be taken into consideration, when mining for knowledge discovery on factors affecting tinnitus diagnosis and treatment. As a result, additional 161 columns were developed for each separate medical state (for example "anxiety", "asthma", "insomnia", "ulcers", etc.). As *Application* is a text column, it was necessary to perform some text manipulation (tokenization) with the use of PL/SQL procedures. Also, problems of misspellings and the same diseases stated in different words, had to be addressed. Some initially derived columns were, thus, merged into a single column, as in example shown in the listing below.

Listing 6.1 Sample COALESCE (merge) operations for disease feature development.
```
1  COALESCE([allergic conjunctivitis],[allergic rhinitis],
2  [allergies]) AS allergic,
3  COALESCE([angina],[angina pectoris]) AS angin,
4  COALESCE([hypetension],[hyptension],[hyper tension],
5  [hypertension], [elevated intraocular hypertension],
6  [ocualr hypertension],[ocular hypertension], [hyertension])
7  as hyper_tension
```

Reasoning behind using "application" features besides "medication" is, there are more pharmaceuticals that can be used for the same purpose (for example, for an application described as "depression" several medications can be prescribed, including Prozac, Xanax, etc.). Therefore, application features provide more generalization and less selectivity than medication features. They can also be useful for the purpose of experiments on rule extraction.

Two other features were retained from *Pharmacology* table—each patient was denoted with True/False information in *T side* bit column, which informs whether tinnitus is associated with the pharmaceuticals. Also attribute *MedNr* was created that informs how many different medication a patient was taking at the time of diagnosis and treatment start.

Using this approach maximal informational content from pharmacology was retained, having, at the same time, data format more suitable for building more reliable classification model. Some information was left out, however, so that to simplify assumptions for now. For instance, information about dosing (quantitative use of medications), as well as the time period for which the medication had been taken (*Duration*), was omitted. According to our medical expertise, there are basically two types of information in this table: (1) a drug, which can have different names and (2) for what it is prescribed. It is possible to extract information about categories of drugs, e.g., SSRI, benzodiazepines, antibiotics which actually can be more informative than analyzing individual drugs.

6.3.3 Experiment Results

The resulting dataset contained 3125 tuples described by the features (including medication columns) or 603 features (including additionally application of medication columns). Dimension of input matrix changed, in comparison to the previous experimental setup (of 6991 instances and 161 features). This time also *DOB* and *Zip* columns were excluded from building a classifier, as they can overestimate accuracy (by relating visits of the same patient). The model built with J48 (C4.5 tree algorithm in WEKA) was evaluated with 69.7% accuracy (and F-measure of 0.68) for the first mentioned dataset, and 70.2% accuracy (F-measure 0.69) for the extended dataset. Most numerous confusions were that of patients with "1" category classified as "2" category, and C-3 patients classified as C-1 patients. Chi-squared ranker pointed: *P* (problem), *AgeInd* (age when problem was induced), *AgeBeg* (age when treatment started), and *Th R, Th L* (audiological measurements) as the most relevant features. Therefore, there is still a supposition that classification was based on patient's identifiable information that is repeated with each visit.

6.4 One-Patient-One-Tuple Experiment

Another dataset was prepared so that to contain initial visits only (numbered as "0" or "1"), that is, when diagnosis is performed and course of treatment decided. Such dataset consists of 1090 tuples (the number of patients doubles approximately because most of them have these two first visits in the database)- about one third of the dataset with all visits, but the problem with potential information leakage between training and testing data is alleviated. Classification results with J48 model was 52,11% correctly classified instances (which is not that good). Nevertheless, there was still repetitive data, as the dataset contained both "0" and "1" visits (one patient data could be repeated twice).

When considering dataset containing visits numbered as "0" only (so that each tuple represented distinct patient, as each patient has only one visit "0"), dataset was reduced to 599 instances, which is reasonable from medical point of view. The most relevant features, selected with rank method based on chi-squared measure, are shown in Fig. 6.7. It could be observed that the most relevant features in predicting patient's tinnitus category are audiological measurements. According to our medical expertise, these are the most reliable results and some of measurements are expected to be highly correlated, e.g., average threshold of hearing with MLL and MRR and with threshold of white noise.

Chi-squared Ranking Filter

Ranked attributes:

725.05001	45 LR4
712.70417	29 Th L
688.00398	44 LR3
683.38374	43 LR2
683.09068	42 LR1
672.58042	23 T LR
670.57001	47 LR8
667.46635	52 LL3
618.93623	24 Th R
617.06273	51 LL2
606.21401	53 LL4
603.4837	50 LL1
589.86863	55 LL8
585.03241	54 LL6
581.71272	46 LR6
573.40413	49 LL50
572.54551	28 T LL
553.86731	48 LR12
534.10423	41 LR50
527.04316	116 P
493.95612	86 Prob
480.98386	56 LL12
474.4102	31 WNR
455.47575	32 WNL
410.45686	4 R2
393.19923	37 MLL
387.73904	33 MRR

Fig. 6.7 Attributes ranking based on chi-squared measure for dataset with initial visits only

In cross-validation process instances were predicted with 53.4% accuracy with Random Forest, 52% with Naive Bayes and 41.4% with J48 (without feature selection, on 603 attributes). After applying feature selection the accuracy improved, especially for the Naive Bayes classifier—the best result—57.43% was obtained with about 100 features. After increasing number of features beyond 100, the accuracy was decreasing for this algorithm. The details on class distribution in the dataset and results for different categories are shown in Figs. 6.8 and 6.9.

The smallest number of patients was available for category 4. Consequently, the classification results on this category were the worst. The most frequent were patient with "1" and "2" category (177 and 136 correspondingly, out of 599), and these categories were, therefore, predicted with best F-score (precision and recall) and TP/FP rates.

Tree-based classifiers after calibration (using different feature selection) performed: J48 about 43.2% and Random Forest about 51% correctly classified instances, with feature selection set at about 50 attributes. These are still very low results, from medical point of view.

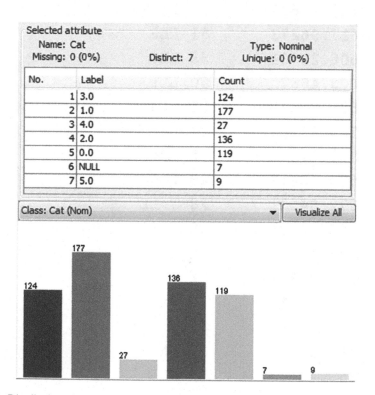

Fig. 6.8 Distribution of category values in training data containing initial visits

=== Detailed Accuracy By Class ===

TP Rate	FP Rate	Precision	Recall	F-Measure	ROC Area	Class
0.613	0.101	0.613	0.613	0.613	0.889	3.0
0.695	0.178	0.621	0.695	0.656	0.843	1.0
0.111	0.016	0.25	0.111	0.154	0.789	4.0
0.721	0.119	0.641	0.721	0.678	0.898	2.0
0.37	0.142	0.393	0.37	0.381	0.711	0.0
0	0	0	0	0	0.815	NULL
0	0	0	0	0	0.444	5.0
Weighted Avg. 0.574	0.129	0.545	0.574	0.557	0.83	

=== Confusion Matrix ===

```
  a   b   c   d   e   f   g   <-- classified as
 76  17   7  13  11   0   0 |   a = 3.0
  8 123   0  16  30   0   0 |   b = 1.0
 13   3   3   4   4   0   0 |   c = 4.0
  5  11   1  98  21   0   0 |   d = 2.0
 17  39   1  18  44   0   0 |   e = 0.0
  1   2   0   3   1   0   0 |   f = NULL
  4   3   0   1   1   0   0 |   g = 5.0
```

Fig. 6.9 Naive Bayes (with 100 selected features) prediction results for each category

6.5 Summary of Classification Experiments

The initial experiments on the dataset containing repetitive data brought optimistic results, which were, however, not reliable (due to cross-validation method and lack of new data for testing). Also, features selected for classification were unsuitable, as they were based on patient's identifiable information, such as date of birth, Zip code of address, which should not affect decision on diagnosis. Such approach indicates potential procedural problem.

Experiments on dataset containing only initial visits, used for categorization only, with medications and their applications developed as pivotal features, brought the most reliable results, because each object was represented by different patient (although the best accuracy was about 57%). The best classifier is based on Naive Bayes and takes only subset of features (ranked based on chi-squared measure) into account (about 1/6 of original number of attributes). The chosen features are mostly based on audiological measures, which is a common-sense approach for performing tinnitus diagnosis (see Table 6.2).

There is a need for further dataset preprocessing and feature development, so that to retain 'object as a patient' dataset model, but, on the other hand, include information from visits other than initial (and develop them into temporal features), which can provide more insight into tinnitus diagnosis and treatment methodology. From medical point of view, treatment depends on classification of patients, and results of treatment could be related to correctness of categorization.

Table 6.2 Summary of experiments' classification accuracy with different preprocessing (dataset structure), feature selection and algorithm

Object represented as	Instances	Features	J48 %	Naive Bayes %	Random forest %
Patient-visit-medication	6991	80	88.5	75.2	89.3
Patient-visit-medication	6991	20	87.9	81.5	87.1
Patient-visit	3125	603	70.2	55.4	71
Patient-visit	3125	488	69.7		
Patient-visit0v1	1090	603	52.11	46	49.2
Patient-visit0	599	603	43.2	52	53.4
Patient-visit0	599	100	41	57.4	49.5

A general conclusion is that too many attribute values in the dataset are missing (for example, there is no demographic information of patients from years 2004–2005 at all, and no pharmacology data for patients from 2005).

6.5.1 Final Classifier Choice

When implementing into recommender system, the prediction model built on initial visits only (Patient-Visit0 data model) with Naive Bayes algorithm and feature selection would be considered. The classifier is based mostly on audiological measures, but also on Newman forms answers, some demographics information and number of medications taken. Therefore, it would be sufficient to collect this information when using computer system in supporting diagnosis.

Based on diagnosed tinnitus category, different treatment approach is taken (see table on TRT protocol—2.1). The classifier could be useful especially for differentiating between 1-, 2- and 3-category patients (the best results were obtained for these categories).

Classifiers with accuracy about 50% can be also implemented for testing purposes on new patients' data cases. In order to improve classification additional features should be developed, based on temporal characteristics of consecutive visits.

Chapter 7
Experiment 2: Diagnostic Rules

Abstract Association rule tasks were defined in order to discover common patterns in patients' visits dataset. Before defining data mining task on rule discovery, it is necessary to formulate an analytical problem in the first place. The main examined associations of interest would be factors affecting patient's category. Such discovered association rules can be regarded as decision rules, supporting classifier developed in the previous step.

7.1 Methodology

Process of diagnosis and determining patient's category, in terms of data flow and affecting factors, was examined once again. The basic protocol is shown in Fig. 7.1. This schema is much simplified as, for example, interview is providing much more information than demographic, which is at best secondary and basically collected for formal reasons.

An initial visit, when a problem is determined, consists of following subprocesses (as described in [JJ00]):

- initial contact with the patient (form is sent by mail to individuals interested to be treated in the center),
- interview, being an expansion of form responses,
- audiological evaluation (otoscopic evaluation and series of tests, from which a basic audiogram with LDLs is crucial),
- medical evaluation (identifying medical conditions that may cause, contribute to, or have an impact on the treatment of tinnitus),
- diagnosis with decision regarding the treatment category (patient is placed into one of five categories Fig. 2.1).

Analysis of the process and data flow leads to conclusion that it would be sensible to search for relations between:

K.A. Tarnowska et al., *Decision Support System for Diagnosis and Treatment of Hearing Disorders*, Studies in Computational Intelligence 685,
DOI 10.1007/978-3-319-51463-5_7

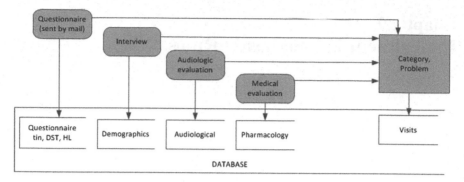

Fig. 7.1 Factors and data flow in the process of determining patient's category and problem

- audiological measurements,
- demographics/form data,
- pharmacology (except for pharmacology which is not used for categorization),

and patient's category. All these factors take part in the diagnosis process and help physician to determine a problem and category of a patient and then follow a suitable protocol of treatment. The treatment approach varies according to category; thus, accurate placement of patients into these categories is critical to provide proper treatment.

Experiments on diagnostic rule discovery (association rules) were carried out with LISp-Miner system, which offers exploratory data analysis, implemented by its own procedures, called GUHA. The LISp-Miner system is an academic system used mainly for data mining research and teaching. It is being developed at University of Economics in Prague since 1996. Currently LISp-Miner consists of ten data min-

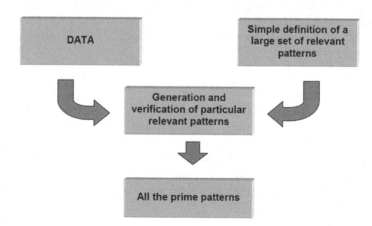

Fig. 7.2 GUHA method in LISp-Miner rule discovery [Nek]

object i.e. row of $\mathcal{M}$	columns of $\mathcal{M}$ i.e. attributes				examples of literals	
	A_1	A_2	...	A_{50}	$A_1(1,2)$	$\neg A_{50}(6)$
o_1	1	4	...	4	T	T
o_2	4	3	...	6	F	F
o_3	2	6	...	7	T	T
$\vdots$	$\vdots$	$\vdots$	$\ddots$	$\vdots$	$\vdots$	$\vdots$
o_n	3	1	...	36	F	T

Fig. 7.3 Bit-string approach to mine association rules [Nek]

ing analytical procedures plus thirteen other modules supporting e.g. the *Business understanding* and *Data preprocessing* phases of the data mining process [Sim14].

4 ft-Miner module of LISp-Miner system was used for association rules discovery and Ac4ft-Miner for action rules. The GUHA method, an original Czech data-mining method with strong theoretical background, uses definition of the set of association rules (or G-rules in Ac4ft-Miner) to generate and verify particular rules on the data provided to the system (see Fig. 7.2). The algorithm is highly optimized to generate results in a reasonable time [Sim14].

Algorithm does not use Apriori-like, but bit-string approach to mine rules. As depicted on Fig. 7.3, input data matrix of nominal attributes is converted into boolean attributes (literals). Antecedent and consequent of the GUHA rule (relevant pattern) are defined in terms of boolean attributes, which are, in turn, defined as conjunction or disjunction of boolean attributes or literals.

7.1.1 Data Source

Data input for LISp-Miner is a data matrix created by *LMDataSource* module. The data matrix is created from one database table. The input matrix is transformed into format readable by the system's procedure, as described in the previous section.

For the purpose of the following experiments, the ODBC connection to the source database was configured, so that SQL preprocessing operations can be performed flexibly on the data and become available to *LMDataSource* module. The dataset for preliminary experiments consists of patient's visits, with medications and diseases developed as pivotal features (3 125 tuples described by about 600 features). Attribute definition and data preparation step is discussed in more detail in the next section.

Table 7.1 Tinnitus patients' and visits' attributes definition in LISp-Miner

Group	Att name	Attribute meaning	Type	Cat	Sample
General	THC	Patient identifier	Nom	583	00001
	V	Visit number	Nom	36	0, 1, 2, 3, 4
	P	Problems in order	Nom	15	H, HLT, TL
	Miso	Misophonia	Nom	2	Yes/no
	Miso treat	Miso treatment protocol	Nom	4	1, 2, 3, 4
	FU	Follow-up contact	Nom	5	A, C, T, E
	DP	Dependency of H presence	Nom	2	Yes/no
	REM	Real-ear measurements	Nom	2	Yes/no
	C	Category assigned by doctor	Nom	6	0, 1, 2, 3, 4
	CC	Category chosen by patient	Nom	6	0,1, 2, 3, 4
Audiological	R25	RE pure-tone thresh 0.25 kHz	Inter	8	$<-10;0)$
	R50	RE pure-tone thresh 0.50 kHz	Inter	8	$<-5;0)$
	...	...	...	...	...
	L25	LE pure-tone thresh 0.25 kHz	Inter	8	$<-5;0)$
	...	...	...	...	...
	LR50	Loudness Discomfort Level R	Inter	8	$<12;75)$
	LL50	Loudness Discomfort Level L	Inter	8	$<11;77)$
	...	...	...	...	...
	T PR	T pitch match	Inter	40	$<0.35;1)$
	T Rm	RE match type	Nom	4	NB, NBN
	T LR	T loudness match dB	Inter	4	$<4;22)$
	Th R	RE threshold of hearing	Inter	50	$<-10;-2)$
	MRR	RE minimal masking level	Inter	8	$<0;26)$
	...	...	...	...	...
Demographics	AgeBeg	Age when treatment began	Inter	7	$<8;40)$
	G	Gender	Nom	2	f/m
	Occup	Occupation	Nom	54	Engineer
	Work	Work status	Nom	4	h, r, s, w
	MedNr	Number of medications taken	Inter	5	$<1;2)$
	Country	Country of residence	Nom	9	USA, Chile
	State	State of residence	Nom	31	AL, GA
	Zip	Zip code of residence	Nom	181	01742

(continued)

Table 7.1 (continued)

Group	Att name	Attribute meaning	Type	Cat	Sample
Tinnitus	AgeInd	Age problem started	Inter	7	<7;30)
	AATI	Tin induced by auto accident	Nom	2	Yes/no
	DETI	Tin induced by depression	Nom	2	Yes/no
	HLTI	Tin assoc with hearing loss	Nom	2	Yes/no
	NTI	Tin induced by noise	Nom	2	Yes/no
	STI	Tin induced by stress	Nom	2	Yes/no
	OTI	Tin induced by operation	Nom	2	Yes/no
	OMTI	Tin induced by other medical	Nom	2	Yes/no
	T side	Tin as side-effect of pharm	Nom	2	Yes/no
	Gradual	Gradual onset of tinnitus	Nom	2	Yes/no
	Sudden	Sudden onset of tinnitus	Nom	2	Yes/no
Condition	Aches	Aches present?	Nom	2	Yes/no
	...		...	...	...
	Menieres	Menieres disease present?	Nom	2	Yes/no
	...		...	...	...
	Vertigo	Vertigo present?	Nom	2	Yes/no
Medication	Accupiril	Accupiril taken?	Nom	2	Yes/no
	...		...	...	...
	Zyrtec	Zyrtec taken?	Nom	2	Yes/no
Instruments	Ins	Instrument category	Nom	3	SG, HA
	Type	Type of instrument	Nom	6	GHH
	Model	Model of instrument	Nom	16	BTE
	Ins vis	Instrument (Visits table)	Nom	43	BTE, GHS
	Instr	Instrument (Question table)	Nom	32	SG, GHS
REM	Freg RE	Right-ear measurements	Inter	12	<39;2000)
	Th R SPL		Inter	25	<22;26)
	Mix R SPL		Inter	25	<4;31)
	Mix R SL		Inter	15	<0;2)
	Tol R SPL		Inter	25	<7;29)
	Tol R SL		Inter	15	<4;8)
	Max R SPL		Inter	25	<43;48)
	Max R SL		Inter	25	<6;11)
	Freg LE	Left-ear measurements	Inter	12	<50;2000)
	...		...	...	...

(continued)

Table 7.1 (continued)

Group	Att name	Attribute meaning	Type	Cat	Sample
Interview	An t	% of time when annoyed	Inter	10	<0;2)
	Aw t	% of time when aware	Inter	10	<0;7.5)
	Out	Outcome	Nom	4	B, N, S, W
	T sv	Severity of tinnitus	Inter	5	<0;3)
	T an	Annoyance of tinnitus	Inter	5	<0;3)
	T EL	Tinnitus effect on life	Inter	5	<0;2)
	T pr	Tinnitus as a problem	Inter	5	<0;2.5)
	H pr	Hyperacusis as a problem	Inter	5	<0;0.5)
	HL pr	Hearing loss as a problem	Inter	5	<0;0.5)
	DST	Oversensitivity y/n	Nom	2	Y, N
	Phys	Physical discomfort y/n	Nom	2	Y, N
	Descr	Descr of troublesome sound	Nom	43	Sirens
	Concert	Activity prevented	Nom	5	0, 2, 4
	Shopp	Shopping prevented	Nom	5	0, 2, 4
	Mov	Movies prevented	Nom	5	0, 2, 4
	Wrk	Work prevented	Nom	5	0, 2, 4
	Rest	Restaurants prevented	Nom	5	0, 2, 4
	Drv	Driving prevented	Nom	5	0, 2, 4
	Sport	Sports prevented	Nom	5	0, 2, 4
	Church	Church prevented	Nom	5	0, 2, 4
	House	Housekeeping prevented	Nom	5	0, 2, 4
	Child	Childcare prevented	Nom	5	0, 2, 4
	Soc	Social activities prevented	Nom	5	0, 2, 4
	Oth	Other activities prevented	Nom	5	0, 2, 4
	H sv	Severity of DST	Inter	5	<0;1.5)
	H an	Annoyance of DST	Inter	5	<0;1.5)
	H EL	DST effect on life	Inter	5	<0;1)
	Pr	Program assessment	Nom	3	Y, N, U
	Ret	Returning Instruments	Nom	2	Y, N
NewmanQ	F1	Difficult to concentrate?	Nom	3	0, 2, 4
	F2	Difficult to hear people?	Nom	3	0, 2, 4
	E3	Tin makes you angry?	Nom	3	0, 2, 4
	F4	Tin makes you confused?	Nom	3	0, 2, 4
	C5	Feel desperate?	Nom	3	0, 2, 4
	E6	Complain about your tin?	Nom	3	0, 2, 4

(continued)

Table 7.1 (continued)

Group	Att name	Attribute meaning	Type	Cat	Sample
	F7	Sleeping problems?	Nom	3	0, 2, 4
	C8	Feel cannot escape your tin?	Nom	3	0, 2, 4
	F9	Tin interfere social activities?	Nom	3	0, 2, 4
	E10	Feel frustrated?	Nom	3	0, 2, 4
	C11	Feel have a terrible disease?	Nom	3	0, 2, 4
	F12	Difficult for you to enjoy life?	Nom	3	0, 2, 4
	F13	Job /house responsibilities?	Nom	3	0, 2, 4
	E14	Tin make you often irritable?	Nom	3	0, 2, 4
	F15	Difficult for you to read?	Nom	3	0, 2, 4
	E16	Tinnitus make you upset?	Nom	3	0, 2, 4
	E17	Stress on your relationships?	Nom	3	0, 2, 4
	F18	Difficult to focus attention?	Nom	3	0, 2, 4
	C19	No control over your tinnitus?	Nom	3	0, 2, 4
	F20	Tin makes you often tired?	Nom	3	0, 2, 4
	E21	Tin makes you depressed?	Nom	3	0, 2, 4
	E22	Tinnitus makes you anxious?	Nom	3	0, 2, 4
	C23	Cannot cope with your tin?	Nom	3	0, 2, 4
	F24	Tin worse when under stress?	Nom	3	0, 2, 4
	E25	Tin makes you feel insecure?	Nom	3	0, 2, 4
	Sc F	Total score: Function	Inter	6	<0;6)
	Sc E	Total score: Emotion	Inter	6	<0;4)
	Sc C	Total score: Catastrophic	Inter	6	<0;2)
	Sc T	Total score: sum of above	Inter	5	Mild

7.1.2   Attributes

Preliminary data preparation included creating a primary key column, setting groups of attributes, defining attributes from table columns, and categories from the attribute values.

Table 7.1 shows tinnitus database attributes definition and groups they were divided into. The table presents also the category type, number of resulting categories (attribute values) and sample category for each attribute. Attributes of tinnitus patients and visits were defined as either nominal (*each value—one category*—for categorical, character columns), equifrequency or equidistant intervals (discretization method for integer, decimal or float data types). The former approach for interval construction, equifrequency intervals, considers the distribution of the data and is generated automatically based on frequency calculation and number of categories specified by user. The latter enables user to define categories with fixed interval length.

Category definition additionally allowed to double check data integrity by discovering errors in data values: misspellings, out of range values etc. Such erroneous categories were either left out or joined with the correct category, when this could have been inferred. For example, for *Instruments* attribute, category value denoting *Viennatone* instrument was resulting from joining *V, Vivatone, RVivatone, Vivatne* attribute values.

Attributes in General Group-correspond to main features describing each visit:

- identifier of a patient (first two digits denoting year and three next—an ordering number),
- visit number (initial-0, consecutive—1, 2, 3, etc.),
- problems in order of importance (T-tinnitus, H-hyperacusis, L-hearing loss, M-misophonia),
- attributes related to misophonia (whether fear of sound present in patient and protocol of misophonia treatment followed),
- type of follow-up contact (A-audiology and counseling, C-counseling, T-telephone, E-email, M-Mail),
- dependency of hyperacusis presence *DP*,
- *REM*—whether real-ear measurements were performed at the visit,
- and finally categories assigned to a patient by a doctor (C), and category of treatment chosen by a patient (CC).

Audiological Attributes

Summarize the process of audiological evaluation, which is helpful in separating issues of hearing, tinnitus, hyperacusis and misophonia [JJ00]. It consists of otoscopic examination of the ear canal and tympanic membrane, and series of tests. Routine audiological testing includes an evaluation of pure tone thresholds up to 12 kHz (attributes *R25, R50,... R12* and, corresponding, for left ear—*L25, L50,...*

L12) and word recognition scores, providing an assessment of a patient's hearing and a basis for subsequent tinnitus measurements [JJ00]. Specific tinnitus/hyperacusis measurements consist of:

- pitch matching (*T PR/T PL*),
- loudness matching (*T LR/T LL*),
- the minimal masking levels (*MRR, MRL, MRB* for right ear and *MLR, MLL, MLB* for left ear),
- LDLs (attributes denoted as *LR50, LR1, LR2,..., LR12* and *LL50, LL1, LL2, ..., LL12*).

Pitch and loudness matching provide information useful for counseling, but not for diagnosis. The crucial measurements are those of Loudness Discomfort Level (LDL), using pure tones up to 12 kHz, as well as frequency that corresponds to the tinnitus pitch [JJ00]. Measurements are performed twice, and the second set is recorded in the database.

Demographics Attributes

Correspond to columns from the original tables: *Demographics* and *Misc*. They describe a patient in terms of their age when treatment started, gender, occupation, place of residence, work status, etc., but also number of medications they take for different afflictions.

Tinnitus

Embraces attributes describing induction of tinnitus and hyperacusis problem. These include derived from text columns, boolean features informing whether the problem, as perceived by a patient, was a consequence of stress, noise, medical condition, operation, auto accident injury or depression, whether the problem developed gradually or suddenly, and medication uptake was associated with the onset of tinnitus (*T side*). Development of these features was described in Sects. 6.2.1 and 6.2.2). The group also consists of *AgeInd* attribute, which informs what was the age at the time of tinnitus onset. Alternatively boolean attributes such as Y30, Y20, etc. can be used, which indicate what was the time elapse between problem onset and start of the treatment (see Sect. 6.2.2 for detailed description).

Pharmacology

Next two groups, *Condition* and *Medication*, aggregate information derived from original *Pharmacology* table. These are boolean attributes, informing whether a patient was affected by a particular disease at start of treatment and what medications were taken for these additional afflictions (see Sects. 6.4.1 and 6.4.2 for description of pharmacology features development).

Instrumentation

Other two groups of attributes: *Instruments* and *REM* should be helpful in determining treatment actions that potentially can lead to tinnitus improvement. Such actions might be, for example, changing a sound-generating instrument to a different type or model. Type of instruments was originally registered in three different tables: *Instruments*, *Visits* and *Qustionnaire tin*. *REM* denotes real-ear measurements, which is a method of fitting the instrument, by measuring the sound level produced by sound generators inside of ear canal. This also can be regarded an action taken to improve the state of tinnitus perception.

Interview

Besides causative characteristics of tinnitus, as described by attributes in *Tinnitus* group, another important source of information, related to tinnitus, are initial/follow-up forms. They were designed to track the treatment progress and were filled by provider during structured interview with patients at initial/follow-up visits. Forms' structure, presented in appendix A and B, is reflected in suitable attributes, such as:

- percentage of tinnitus awareness/annoyance (*Aw t, An t*),
- tinnitus/ decreased sound tolerance subjective ranked loudness (*T sv/H sv*),
- annoyance and effect on life (on average over last month in 0–10 scale)—*T an, T EL, H an, H EL,*
- activities prevented as a result of sound oversensitivity: concerts, housekeeping, childcare, etc. (expressed in 0–4 scale, 0 meaning no problem).

The *Interview* group also consists of attributes related to tinnitus, hyperacusis, and hearing loss as a problem (average over last month in 0–10 scale)—*T pr, H pr, HL pr*. Besides, patients were asked whether they were glad that they had started the program (*Pr*) and whether they would have considered giving back the instruments (*Ret*). Other columns reflecting form structure consisted of too many missing values to be included in the data mining tasks.

NewmanQ

Groups attributes related to form (*Newman questionnaire*, also named *Tinnitus Handicap Inventory*) consisting of 25 questions, each to be answered on three levels Likur scale, divided into three groups: functional, emotional and catastrophic. Paper version of the form is presented in Appendix C. Each question makes an attribute with categories 0, 2, 4, "0" denoting "yes", "2"—"sometimes" and "4"—"no". New form, evaluating patients emotions in 0 – 10 scale—(*Tinnitus Functional Index*), was not used as these subscales turned out to be useless and they are not used. The group also includes total scores calculated for each of the three groups of questions, and total score, calculated as sum of these three. Total score attribute is an important measure of initial tinnitus severity and treatment. The attribute was defined with five categories, relating scores to tinnitus severity (according to scale as in Appendix C): 0–16—slight, 18–36—mild, 38–56—moderate, 58–76—severe, and 78–100—catastrophic handicap. The aim of action rule extraction would be to find treatment actions that lead to changes in a patients' tinnitus severity from higher to lower.

Preliminary experiment did not consider temporal dependencies (all data of timestamp type was not used in the preliminary experiments). It means that each consecutive visit was considered to be of the same time elapse from the previous one. The same assumption applies to changes in tinnitus indicators (they were not related temporally to previous values).

7.1.3 Tasks Definition

To define a task in 4 ft-Miner module in LISp-Miner it is necessary to define a relevant pattern (as depicted in Fig. 7.2), by setting up:

- antecedent,
- succedent,
- quantifier.

Optionally *condition* can also be specified. For *antecedent* part all attributes, whose result on interesting factor in *succecedent* part will be examined, were chosen. For example, it might be worth checking association between audiological measurements and category of a patient. According to our medical knowledge, it has to be related as categories are defined mainly on the basis of audiological findings, additionally with severity determined by THI. *Quantifier* setting enables to control rule generation. LISp-Miner provides for different types of quantifiers and their settings (for example—implications, equality relations). Formally, a *quantifier* is defined as depicted in Table 7.2.

Confidence

$$Conf = \frac{a}{a+b}$$

Support

$$Supp = \frac{a}{a+b+c+d}$$

Table 7.2 4 ft quantifier: $\phi \implies \psi$, ϕ antecedent, ψ succedent, $\implies$ quantifier

	ψ	$\neg\psi$
ϕ	a	b
$\neg\phi$	c	d

Quantifier

$$\phi \implies_{BASE,p} \psi, \frac{a}{a+b} > p \wedge a \geq BASE$$

Two, default, quantifier settings used in experiments are:

- *BASE*—at least BASE-number of objects is statistically relevant.
- *FUI—Founded implication quantifier*—assuring that at least p * 100% objects satisfying antecedent, satisfy also succedent.

BASE and *FUI* p parameters were adjusted for different runs so that to obtain the best confidence and support, but also taking into account characteristics of the pattern checked (for example, taking into account number of missing values for particular attributes or decision's attribute relative frequency). Standard minimum starting point for the p parameter was 0.5 (it is assumed that rules with confidence lower than 50% cannot be successfully applied in RECTIN). *BASE* quantifier settings ranged from 10 to 80 (when the task generated no hypotheses, *BASE* was lowered).

Conditional Quantifier

$\phi \implies \psi / Condition$ On the grounds that diagnosis is performed at an initial visit, all rules were set with condition on *Visit number* attribute, defined as *one category* coefficient type, set to "0".

Minimum and Maximum Lengths

When setting up a particular task, it is also possible to define the minimum and maximum number of cedents/literals for antecedent and succedent parts.

Cedents

The cedents are chosen from previously defined attributes (in Table 7.1), and for each attribute, following settings are chosen in the task definition:

- coefficient type—for example: subset, one category, sequence, cut, etc.,
- coefficient length—minimum and maximum length,
- gace type: positive, negative, both.

7.2 Results

After setting up a data mining task in LISp-Miner, *Run* option starts GUHA procedure (see Fig. 7.2), and after some time, depending on the task complexity, set of *prime patterns* generated in form of *hypotheses* appears on the output screen. Each hypothesis can be then evaluated in details, with all metrics related to GUHA procedure. In the listings below, only confidence and support values are provided for each rule.

7.2.1 Interview ⟹ Category

Considering that RECTIN system, as depicted in Fig. 5.2, assumes automation in patients' categorization after filling in electronic versions of initial/follow-up forms and performing audiological measurements, it would be useful to discover rules relating form's responses to the corresponding categorization, decided by a doctor. 4 ft-Miner task was set up so that to include attributes from *Interview* group in the antecedent part of relevant pattern. Results from the experiment are shown as examples of obtained hypotheses, in division for particular categories.

Hypotheses 1 $H\,EL < 1 \implies_{0.52;0.04} C(0)$
$H\,An < 1.5 \wedge H\,EL < 1 \wedge H\,Sv < 1.5 \implies_{0.51;0.03} C(0)$

Hypotheses 2 $HL\,pr < 0.5 \wedge T\,EL \geq 8 \implies_{0.55;0.06} C(1)$
$H\,pr < 0.5 \wedge HL\,pr < 0.5 \implies_{0.58;0.04} C(1)$

Hypotheses 3 $HL\,pr \geq 5 \wedge T\,EL \geq 8 \implies_{0.57;0.07} C(2)$
$HL\,pr \geq 5 \wedge T\,Sv \geq 8 \implies_{0.57;0.06} C(2)$
$HL\,pr \geq 5 \wedge T\,An \geq 8 \implies_{0.55;0.07} C(2)$
$HL\,pr \geq 5 \implies_{0.54;0.016} C(2)$
$HL\,pr \geq 5 \wedge T\,Pr \geq 8 \implies_{0.52;0.06} C(2)$

Hypotheses 4 $H\,An \geq 8 \wedge H\,EL \geq 8 \wedge H\,Sv \geq 7.5 \implies_{0.58;0.09} C(3)$
$H\,pr \geq 7 \wedge H\,An \geq 8 \wedge H\,EL \geq 8 \wedge H\,Sv \geq 7.5 \implies_{0.58;0.08} C(3)$

The obtained rules confirm the expert (medical) knowledge (compare with Table 2.1):

- patients categorized into 0 group have a problem with low impact on life ($H\,EL$ is low),
- category-1 patients have significant tinnitus problem, but without hyperacusis ($H\,pr$ is low) and there is no significant hearing loss ($HL\,pr$ is low),
- category 2 is characterized on the other hand with significant hearing loss ($HL\,pr \geq 5$),
- category 3 is associated by the expert with significant hyperacusis problem [MLDK10]—obtained hypotheses show association of high values of $H\,An$, $H\,Sv$ and $H\,EL$ with this category.

7.2.2 Audiology ⟹ Category

Second 4 ft-Miner task was designed to find dependencies, in form of association rules, between audiological measurements and category of a patient, deter-

mined by a doctor. Antecedents were set to attributes from *Audiological* group
(defined as equifrequent intervals). Succedent part was set to each of patient category, subsequently—0, 1, 2, 3 and 4 (coefficient type for *C* attribute was set as *One
category*). Examples of generated association rules, for each of the category, with
the corresponding confidence and support values are shown as hypotheses below.

Hypotheses 5 $LSD \geq 100 \wedge LL4 \geq 999 \wedge LR8 \geq 999 \wedge RSD \geq 100 \implies_{0.5;0.04} C(0)$
$LSD \geq 100 \wedge LL4 \geq 999 \wedge LL8 \geq 999 \wedge LR8 \geq 999 \wedge RSD \geq 100 \implies_{0.5;0.04} C(0)$

Hypotheses 6 $LL12 \geq 999 \wedge LR12 \geq 999 \wedge RSD \geq 100 \implies_{0.58;0.11} C(1)$
$LL12 \geq 999 \wedge RSD \geq 100 \implies_{0.55;0.12} C(1)$

Hypotheses 7 $LR8 \geq 999 \wedge R4 \geq 65 \implies_{0.78;0.08} C(2)$
$L2 \geq 50 \implies_{0.7;0.1} C(2)$
$R4 \geq 65 \implies_{0.66;0.1} C(2)$

Hypotheses 8 $LR6 < 78 \implies_{0.63;0.07} C(3)$
$LR2 < 74 \implies_{0.62;0.07} C(3)$
$LR1 < 74 \implies_{0.61;0.07} C(3)$
$LL4 < 76 \implies_{0.58;0.07} C(3)$

Hypotheses 9 $LSD \geq 100 \wedge L4 < 10 \; AND \; LL3 < 75 \implies_{0.67;0.02} C(4)$
$L3 < 5 \wedge LL3 < 75 \implies_{0.59;0.02} C(4)$
$L4 < 10 \wedge LL3 < 75 \implies_{0.53;0.02} C(4)$

Rules with best support were obtained for the most numerous categories. Generated hypotheses should be confronted with the expert knowledge, however they
seem to confirm the knowledge as described in medical papers on tinnitus [JJ00].
These say that a basic audiogram with LDLs is the crucial test for diagnosis. The normal LDLs oscillate at about 90–110 dB, 102 being the normal average. The lower the
level, the more decreased sound tolerance with 81.7 dB being the average for patients
with decreased sound tolerance. Based on obtained rules, it can be concluded that
the lower the tolerance, the more severe category of tinnitus should be assigned to a
patient. From medical point of view, the results are interesting and strong correlation
of THI with LDL is expected to some extent in theory.

7.2.3 *Demographics* $\implies$ *Category*

In the next experiment antecedent part was set to literals formed from attributes from
Demographics group, succedent—to patient's category.

Hypotheses 10 *Country(USA)* $\wedge$ *MedNr(<3;4))* $\wedge$ *State(GA)* $\implies_{0.56;0.02} C(0)$

Hypotheses 11 *AgeBeg(<50;55))* $\wedge$ *Country(USA)* $\wedge$ *G(m)* $\implies_{0.58;0.02} C(1)$
AgeBeg(<50;55)) $\wedge$ *G(m)* $\implies_{0.56;0.02} C(1)$
Country(USA) $\wedge$ *G(m)* $\wedge$ *M6(yes)* $\implies_{0.5;0.02} C(1)$

Hypotheses 12 $AgeBeg \geq 68 \implies_{0.58;0.03} C(2)$
$AgeBeg \geq 68 \wedge Country(USA) \implies_{0.58;0.03} C(2)$
$G(m) \wedge MedNr \geq 5 \implies_{0.55;0.03} C(2)$
$G(m) \wedge MedNr \geq 5 \wedge T\,side(yes) \implies_{0.53;0.03} C(2)$

Hypotheses 13 $Work(h) \implies_{0.69;0.02} C(3)$
$Work(h) \wedge T\,side(yes) \implies_{0.67;0.01} C(3)$
$Country(USA) \wedge G(f) \wedge M1(yes) \implies_{0.83;0.01} C(3)$
$AgeBeg \geq 40 \wedge Country(USA) \wedge AgeInd(<30;38)) \implies_{0.71;0.01} C(3)$
$Occup(homemaker) \implies_{0.71;0.01} C(3)$
$G(f) \wedge STI(yes) \implies_{0.5;0.01} C(3)$

Hypotheses 14 $Country(USA) \wedge G(m) \wedge MedNr(3) \wedge Y10(yes) \implies_{0.8;0.01} C(4)$

Some relevant patterns of patients' demographics in particular categories were found out. For example, as a rule, patients with tinnitus of low effect on life (that is 0-category) came from Georgia state in the USA (that is nearby the clinic) and were affected with 3 other afflictions (took 3 medications for treating them). Confronting these results with medical expertise, it might just reflect the fact that long distance patients with low level of severity did not bother to come as it would involve cost and effort; coming was much easier for people from Georgia.

Common pattern for patients in category 1 was: a male aged 50–55 from the USA, whose tinnitus had started 6–12 months before he began TRT.

It could be also observed that category-2 patients are typically older (age when began treatment typically higher than 68 years old as a rule), they had taken more medication (5 and more) and their tinnitus was associated with taking these medications (*T side(yes)*). Medical experience shows that older patients are taking more medications. Also, hearing loss, which has to be present for Category 2, is strongly correlated with age.

Relevant patterns for category 3 included:

- patients who worked at home (and also they tinnitus was induced by medications),
- patients occupied with homemaking,
- patients who were females with tinnitus induced 1–3 months before they went to a doctor,
- females whose tinnitus was associated with stressful situations,
- patients relatively young (younger than 40 years old, whose problem started at 30–38 years old), living in the USA.

Pattern found for patients with most severe, fourth category, included males curing three other afflictions with medications, whose tinnitus is 10–20 years old.

It should be noted that these rules must not be primarily used in diagnosis. Patient's category should not be based on their age, place of residence, occupation, etc., but rather on more objective factors, from medical point of view, such as, audiological measures or interview. Nevertheless, they reveal some common demographic patterns in categories of patients treated in the past, which may bring additional knowledge, used as heuristics or hints.

7.2.4 Pharmacology $\Longrightarrow$ Category

Next experiments were focused on discovering patterns relating additional patients' afflictions and medication taken in order to cure them, to the category of tinnitus treatment. Preliminary results have shown that patients with accompanying depression, anxiety or panic disorders were assigned to category 1, while patients with hypertension, for example, belonged to category 2.

Hypotheses 15 *Ativan(yes)* $\wedge$ *Anxiety disorder(yes)* $\Longrightarrow$ $_{0.58;0.01}$ *C(1)*
Klonopin(yes) $\wedge$ *Panic disorder(yes)* $\wedge$ *Seizures(yes)* $\Longrightarrow$ $_{0.53;0.01}$ *C(1)*
Depression disorder(yes) $\wedge$ *Panic disorder(yes)* $\wedge$ *Seizures(yes)* $\Longrightarrow$ $_{0.5;0.02}$ *C(1)*

Relevant group of patients treated for anxiety, panic/seizures or depression disorders (with Ativan/Klonopin) was diagnosed with the first category of tinnitus. These drugs are routinely prescribed by physicians in case of tinnitus, to decrease anxiety or depression.

Hypotheses 16 *Angin(yes)* $\wedge$ *Hypertension(yes)* $\Longrightarrow$ $_{0.69;0.02}$ *C(2)*

Patients with hypertension and angina can be hypothetically classified into second category of tinnitus (with 69% confidence). According to medical expertise, typically these conditions are associated with aging which in turn is strongly associated with hearing loss.

Hypotheses 17 *Premarin(yes)* $\wedge$ *Menopause(yes)* $\wedge$ *Vulval anthropy(yes)* $\Longrightarrow$ $_{0.55;0.01}$ *C(3)*

Patients (females) with menopause, treated with Premarin, are associated with tinnitus category 3 (with 55% confidence). These results are interesting from medical point of view, as there are physiological mechanisms linking tinnitus and hyperacusis with sex hormones.

7.2.5 Age $\Longrightarrow$ Diseases

To provide more insightful conclusions on association between age, medical condition and tinnitus category, relation between age and diseases was examined.

Hypotheses 18 *AgeBeg(<40;45))* $\Longrightarrow$ $_{0.63;0.03}$ *Depression disorder(yes)*
AgeBeg $\geq$ *68* $\Longrightarrow$ $_{0.48;0.03}$ *Hypertension(yes)*

It seems that depression as a rule existed in tinnitus patients at age between 40 and 45 with 63% confidence, while hypertension in patients older than 68 years. The latter age group was also, most often, associated with category 2 of tinnitus (see Hypotheses 12), and this category was also, hypothetically, associated with hypertension (see Hypotheses 16). Therefore, both experiments are consistent in their results.

This additional insight into medical condition of patients, beside their demographics, confirms that category 1 was more typical for middle-aged patients and associated with depression, anxiety disorders and their tinnitus could have had more psychological background. On the other hand, patients from category 2, that is, more elderly patients (as previous experiments have shown), were treated for old-age-related diseases such as hypertension, diabetes, arthritis, which are also associated with category 2. Some of these patients also took medications for their angina. Category 3 included significant number of women treated for menopause, which could be also perceived as a stressful situation in life (females and stress was associated with this category in previous experiments—see Hypotheses 13). When confronted with medical knowledge, however, it might be more direct physiological link, as stress is prevalent in all categories and patients.

7.2.6 Pharmacology $\implies$ Tinnitus

The following experiment was conducted to discover pharmaceuticals that may most commonly contribute to the tinnitus onset. The corresponding task was defined in such a way, so that partial cedent on *T side* attribute (tinnitus as a side-effect of medications) was defined with coefficient as *One category* set to "yes". The results are shown as hypotheses below.

Hypotheses 19 *Norvasc(yes)* $\wedge$ *T side(yes)* $\implies$ $_{0.67;0.01}$ *C(2)*
Prozac(yes) $\wedge$ *T side(yes)* $\implies$ $_{0.6;0.01}$ *C(1)*
Synthroid(yes) $\wedge$ *T side(yes)* $\implies$ $_{0.6;0.01}$ *C(2)*
Atenolol(yes) $\wedge$ *T side(yes)* $\implies$ $_{0.56;0.01}$ *C(2)*
Celebrex(yes) $\wedge$ *T side(yes)* $\implies$ $_{0.56;0.01}$ *C(2)*
Klonopin(yes) $\wedge$ *T side(yes)* $\implies$ $_{0.56;0.01}$ *C(1)*

The first medication is applied for hypertension and angina, the second for depression, bulimia nervosa, OCD. Synthroid is used in thyroid hormone therapy, Atenolol reduces blood pressure (treats hypertension). Celebrex acts anti-inflammatory and Klonopin—anti-panic and anti-seizure.

The conclusion from the experiment is that these medications should be further investigated on their side-effects. Patients taking them and seeking help for their tinnitus might recover simply after stop taking them or switching to another complementary pharmaceuticals, with no such side-effects. It might also save time on complex tinnitus therapy, avoiding unnecessary actions. As for depression, however, it is not clear, whether this disorder is cause or effect of tinnitus. From medical point of view, it can be both.

7.2.7 Comprehensive Decision Rules

Last experiment on association rules combines all factors influencing tinnitus diagnosis decision at an initial visit (as depicted in Fig. 7.1), so that to obtain the best decision rules for each category. The sets of rules were divided into the best, in terms of confidence, and the best, in terms of support. These obtained from experiments targeting the best confidence can be interpreted as being more accurate, but less general. On the other hand, rules extracted with settings, so that to obtain best support, held true more generally (in greater populations). It can be noticed that rules with greater confidence, but relatively lower support, are more specific, in terms of their antecedents (have more literals in the antecedent part), while rules with relatively greater support need less premises to arrive at their conclusions. The latter fact might be useful, when new patient's data is incomplete or only partial information, about them, is available.

Most General

Hypotheses 20 $H\,EL < 1 \implies_{0.52;0.04} C(0)$
$L\,SD \geq 100 \wedge LL4 \geq 999 \wedge LR8 \geq 999 \wedge R\,SD \geq 100 \implies_{0.5;0.04} C(0)$
$L\,SD \geq 100 \wedge LL4 \geq 999 \wedge LL8 \geq 999 \wedge LR8 \geq 999 \wedge R\,SD \geq 100 \implies_{0.5;0.04} C(0)$

Hypotheses 21 $LL12 \geq 999 \wedge LR12 \geq 999 \wedge R\,SD \geq 100 \implies_{0.58;0.11} C(1)$
$LR12 \geq 999 \wedge T\,EL \geq 8 \implies_{0.57;0.09} C(1)$
$T\,An \geq 8 \wedge R\,SD \geq 100 \implies_{0.56;0.09} C(1)$

Hypotheses 22 $L4 \geq 65 \implies_{0.62;0.1} C(2)$
$HL\,pr \geq 5 \implies_{0.54;0.14} C(2)$

Hypotheses 23 $H\,An \geq 8 \wedge H\,Sv \geq 7.5 \implies_{0.55;0.1} C(3)$
$H\,Sv \geq 7.5 \implies_{0.5;0.11} C(3)$
$H\,EL \geq 8 \implies_{0.5;0.11} C(3)$

Hypotheses 24 $L\,SD \geq 100 \wedge L4 < 10 \wedge LL3 < 75 \implies_{0.67;0.02} C(4)$
$L3 < 5 \wedge LL3 < 75 \implies_{0.59;0.02} C(4)$
$L4 < 10 \wedge LL3 < 75 \implies_{0.53;0.02} C(4)$

Most Accurate

Hypotheses 25 $DST(N) \implies_{0.78;0.01} C(0)$
$Concert(0) \implies_{0.75;0.01} C(0)$
$Rest(0) \implies_{0.75;0.01} C(0)$

Hypotheses 26 $R3(<15;20)) \wedge T An \geq 8 \implies {}_{0.94;0.03} C(1)$
$LL2 \geq 999 \wedge LR12 \geq 999 \wedge R4(<15;20)) \wedge T EL \geq 8 \implies {}_{0.94;0.03} C(1)$
$LR12 \geq 999 \wedge R4(<15;20)) \wedge T EL \geq 8 \implies {}_{0.94;0.03} C(1)$
$R4(<15;20)) \wedge T Sv \geq 8 \implies {}_{0.94;0.03} C(1)$

Hypotheses 27 $LR8 \geq 999 \wedge R6 \geq 75 \wedge T Sv \geq 8 \implies {}_{0.96;0.04} C(2)$
$LL8 \geq 999 \wedge LR8 \geq 999 \wedge R6 \geq 75 \wedge T Sv \geq 8 \implies {}_{0.96;0.04} C(2)$
$LR6 \geq 999 \wedge LR8 \geq 999 \wedge R2 \geq 45 \wedge R3 \geq 60 \wedge R6 \geq 75 \implies {}_{0.95;0.03} C(2)$
$LR6 \geq 999 \wedge LR8 \geq 999 \wedge R2 \geq 45 \wedge R4 \geq 65 \wedge R6 \geq 75 \implies {}_{0.95;0.03} C(2)$
$LR6 \geq 999 \wedge LR8 \geq 999 \wedge R2 \geq 45 \wedge R4 \geq 65 \wedge R8 \geq 75 \implies {}_{0.95;0.03} C(2)$
$L2 \geq 50 \wedge L3 \geq 60 \wedge LR8 \geq 999 \wedge R6 \geq 75 \implies {}_{0.95;0.03} C(2)$

Hypotheses 28 $LL3(<85;91)) \wedge H pr \geq 7 \wedge H Sv \geq 7.5 \implies {}_{1;0.03} C(3)$
$LL3(<85;91)) \wedge H An \geq 8 \wedge H EL \geq 8 \wedge H Sv \geq 7.5 \implies {}_{1;0.03} C(3)$
$LL3(<85;91)) \wedge H EL \geq 8 \wedge H Sv \geq 7.5 \implies {}_{1;0.03} C(3)$
$LR1 < 74 \wedge LR2 < 74 \wedge LR6 < 78 \wedge H pr \geq 7 \wedge H An \geq 8 \implies {}_{0.94;0.03} C(3)$

7.3 Conclusions

The most relevant features for automatic categorization are audiological measurements and interview form responses, as the rules associating them to patient's category were evaluated with the best confidence and support. This observation seems to confirm the validity of classifier constructed in experiments described in the previous chapter (based on Naive Bayes—see Fig. 6.9), as well as features selection method (based chi-squared measure, with its results as shown in Fig. 6.7). Resulting knowledge, in the form of decision rules, might complement WEKA classifier in supporting diagnosis decision.

Although relations between other factors and category are more tenuous, demographic patterns of patients in different categories, can provide a novel insight and help to analyze tinnitus/hyperacusis problem from various perspectives. Such rules can be implemented into RECTIN *Rule Engine Module* and serve as additional hints (but no decision rules). General conclusions from the experiments on demographics, age groups and pharmacology in relation to tinnitus category and to each other, are:

- Category 1 of tinnitus (that is, tinnitus being the main problem but neither hearing loss nor hyperacusis present) was characterized by middle-aged patients and their tinnitus seems to have its background in psychological disorders: depression, anxiety, panic. Therefore, it can be hypothesized that this category should be treated the same way depression (or another psychological disorder) is treated—with personalized counseling. Presumably, after treating a psychological disorder tinnitus perception might decrease.
- Elderly patients (68 and higher), on the other hand, affected in many cases by hypertension and other age-related afflictions, have tinnitus with hearing loss

present (category 2). Therefore, it allows to hypothesize that more effective treatment would be based on treating hearing loss problem, for example, with hearing aids instrumentation with instrument fitting. Confronting the results with medical knowledge, the treatment for this category always involves amplification.

- Category 3 of tinnitus provides far less insight than the two categories, mentioned above. On one hand, it seems to exist in the youngest patients group (30–38 years old), but its background is not very easily seen. Some rules indicate patterns related to occupation, type of work, and gender (female), as well as stress as tinnitus background. This category of patients seem not to show noticeable association with medical conditions (except pattern found for some female, age-related afflictions).
- The least knowledge was retrieved for the least common categories: 0 (tinnitus with low impact on life) and 4 (long-term sound exacerbation). As a matter of fact, not many common patterns were found for the patients in these categories, except for individual patterns: of male patients, whose tinnitus was induced between 10–20 years before starting treatment (for category 4), and of patients residing in the state of Georgia (for category 0).

Number of analytical questions, possible to formulate within 4 ft-Miner task, is unlimited and depends on the requirements of RECTIN system user or needs of physician dealing with tinnitus. Experiments presented in this section show only examples of task definition and their corresponding results, in order to introduce further possibilities of applying association rules mining to tinnitus database. Analogous experiments could be conducted with decision attribute (succedent) set as *Problem* attribute, *Total score*, or any other indicator of tinnitus (such as *Aw t, An t, T sv, T EL*) or audiological measurements, which also can serve as indicators of tinnitus severity.

Relatively low support of the obtained rules results from dataset sparsity and correspondingly, many missing values. Missing values in many potentially interesting attributes were problematic for task definition. Quantifier parameters, such as *BASE* or p for *FUI*, had to be set accordingly low. Consequently, confidence and support of generated hypotheses were relatively lower.

Chapter 8
Experiment 3: Treatment Rules

Abstract Action rules should help in choosing treatment actions in the course of Tinnitus Retraining Therapy in subsequent visits. In order to understand the process of treatment and formulate appropriate data mining tasks in LISp-Miner, it is necessary to identify treatments actions taken by the doctor to improve tinnitus/hyperacusis patient's condition.

8.1 Methodology

Figure 8.1 presents a summary of the TRT treatment process and data flow, with indicators for progress tracking.

Treatment actions, in terms of data source attributes, can be understood as:

- Treatment protocol—after doctor's diagnosis, it is left to patient's decision, which treatment protocol will be followed. Each treatment protocol is tight to a particular tinnitus category.
- Type of follow-up contact—this can be sound therapy and counseling.
- Instrument—instrument type, i.e., hearing aid, sound generator (further divided into GHI soft, GH hard, Viennatone, etc.) or combined, and particular model of the instrument.
- REM—real-ear measurements, which is assisting instrument fitting.

On the other side, it is important to indicate attributes that would be suitable for tracking treatment progress and changes. One of such attributes, naturally, could be *Total score* from *NewmanQ* group. Problem with the attribute is that it is not complete, with about 48.3% values missing. Another candidate for decision attribute would be *Problem* attribute, which is registered separately for each visit and indicates patient's problem in order of importance ("T"-tinnitus, "L"-Hearing loss, "H"-Hyperacusis). There are only about 4.6% missing values of this attribute. It is possible

© Springer International Publishing AG 2017

K.A. Tarnowska et al., *Decision Support System for Diagnosis and Treatment of Hearing Disorders*, Studies in Computational Intelligence 685, DOI 10.1007/978-3-319-51463-5_8

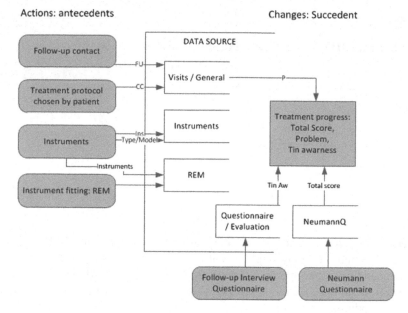

Actions: antecedents   Changes: Succedent

Fig. 8.1 Process and data flow of treatment actions and TRT tracking

to track changes in tinnitus subjective awareness (42.3% missing values), annoyance, tinnitus as a problem (44.6% missing), treatment outcome ("better", "worse", "the same") or other, similar, indicators from the follow-up form. Also, audiological measurements changes can be tracked towards their normal values, as the treatment progresses.

Ac4ft module of LISp-Miner "mines for rules that express which actions should be performed to improve the defined state" [Nek]. The procedure is an implementation of the GUHA method, which mines for G-rules.

To remind, action rule, as defined by Ras and Wieczorkowska [RW00], suggests a change in behavior that can bring an advantage. It consists of two sets of attributes: stable (denoted below as A) and flexible (B):

$$R: (A_1 = \omega_1) \wedge \ldots \wedge (A_q = \omega_q) \wedge (B_1, (\alpha_1 \to \beta_1)) \wedge \ldots \wedge (B_p, (\alpha_p \to \beta_p)) \implies (D, k_1 \to k_2)$$

Decision attribute is denoted as D, and a desirable change as $k_1 \to k_2$. Support and confidence for action rules are calculated in the following way:

- n—the total number of objects in the database
- $CPL(R)$—the number of objects matching $(\omega_1, \ldots, \omega_q, \alpha_1, \ldots, \alpha_p, k_1)$
- $CPR(R)$—the number of objects matching $(\omega_1, \ldots, \omega_q, \beta_1, \ldots, \beta_p, k_2)$
- $CVR(R)$—the number of objects matching $(\omega_1, \ldots, \omega_q, \alpha_1, \ldots, \alpha_p)$
- $CVR(R)$—the number of objects matching $(\omega_1, \ldots, \omega_q, \beta_1, \ldots, \beta_p)$
- $LeftSup(R) = \frac{CPL(R)}{n}$, $RightSup(R) = \frac{CPR(R)}{n}$
- $Sup(R) = LeftSup(R) = \frac{CPL(R)}{n}$

- $Conf(R) = \frac{CPL(R)}{CVL(R)} * \frac{CPR(R)}{CVR(R)}$

8.1.1 Task Definition

In order to set up a task in Ac4ft module, it is necessary to indicate not only attributes for the antecedent and succedent part, but also for their stable and flexible parts. Moreover, the quantifiers are defined in a different way. Formally, G-rule is defined in Ac4ft module as: $\phi_{St} \wedge \Phi_{Chg} \implies {}^* \psi_{St} \wedge \Psi_{Chg}$, where:

- ϕ_{St}—the stable antecedent (or antecedent stable part),
- Φ_{Chg}—the change of antecedent (or antecedent flexible part),
- ψ_{St}—the stable succedent (or succedent stable part),
- Ψ_{Chg}—the change of succedent (or succedent flexible part),
- $\implies {}^*$—Ac4ft quantifier.

G-rule can be expressed by two 4ft-association rules: rule describing an initial state and rule describing a final state. Rule describing initial state is denoted as:
$R_I : \phi_{St} \wedge I(\Phi_{Chg}) \rightarrow_I \psi_{St} \wedge I(\Psi_{Chg})$, then
$R_I : \phi_I \rightarrow_I \psi_I$

	ψ_I	$\neg\psi_I$
ϕ_I	a_I	b_I
$\neg\phi_I$	c_I	d_I

Analogously, rule describing final state:
$R_F : \phi_{St} \wedge F(\Phi_{Chg}) \rightarrow_F \psi_{St} \wedge F(\Psi_{Chg})$, then
$R_F : \phi_F \rightarrow_F \psi_F$

	ψ_F	$\neg\psi_F$
ϕ_F	a_F	b_F
$\neg\phi_F$	c_F	d_F

Ac4ft quantifier used in the experiments is *Founded implication*: $\implies {}^{F>I}_{q,B_I,B_F}$, defined as:
$\frac{a_F}{a_F+b_F} - \frac{a_I}{a_I+b_I} \geq q \wedge a_I \geq B_I \wedge a_F \geq B_F$, where $1 \geq g \geq 0$, $B_I \geq 0$, $B_F \geq 0$.
B_I and B_F are set as parameters to the task: *a (BASE) before* and *a (BASE) after*.

There are also other possibilities for Ac4ft quantifier's definition (for example equity instead of implication). Example of A4ft task definition in LISp-Miner is depicted in Fig. 8.2.

Similarly, as in 4 ft module, a rule is composed of *cedents* (antecedent, succedent, condition), which are understood as a conjunction or disjunction of literals. *Literal* is a basic boolean attribute or negation of a basic boolean attribute. For each attribute we should define:

- minimum and maximum length of literal,

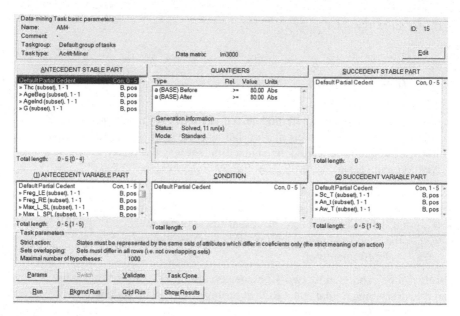

Fig. 8.2 Example definition of a set of relevant rules in Ac4ft mining task

- the type of coefficient—subsets, intervals, left cuts, right cuts, particular value,
- one of the following options: generate only positive literals, only negative, or both.

8.1.2   Decision Attribute Analysis

In approach for action rule extraction, absolute values of total score cannot be used in the succedent flexible part. Such rules would be of low reliability, due to procedure generating them, as simply comparing relative frequency of particular, changeable, features in patients of different tinnitus severity. LISp-Miner algorithm scores action rules based on confidence difference between final and initial state of action. Initial and final state can be satisfied by different patient, who, although can share some features, might be in different stages of treatment (temporal features and dependencies are not considered), their initial tinnitus severity might be different. In summary, such assumptions are too simplified. Consequently, such approach does not consider following contingencies:

- frequency of particular feature can be biased by a total number of a patient's visits and favors patients with higher number of total visits (some features are repeatable with each of the visit),
- approach does not consider changes in a particular patient, instead compares characteristics of patients with different tinnitus severity.

In order to address problems mentioned above, it was decided to implement some additional preprocessing—feature development and missing values imputation. In order to detect actions that in fact brought improvement, another experiment is planned to discover meta-actions, as meta-actions provide the greatest possible treatment personalization. In order to increase efficiency of rule generation, relevant pattern definition should be limited to succedents considering only desirable changes, that is from higher to lower total score category. Thus, additional attribute indicating attribute change was developed, so that to include positive changes only.

8.1.3 Temporal Feature Development

One criterion that is defined by doctor Jastreboff as a "significant improvement" in a patient is [JJ00]: tinnitus awareness decreased by at least 20%, the impact of tinnitus on life decreased by at least 20% and tinnitus annoyance decreased by at least 20%. According to our current medical knowledge, this is an old approach which was used at '90s and which is not used since 2000. The primary criterion is significant change of THI. It has been published that change of 20 points on THI indicated clinically significant improvement.

In order to pursue human approach, additional, derived columns were added to the data source table, so that to relate the current visit's indicator value to the previous value, and therefore, to be able to estimate improvement (or deterioration).

First such derived column—*ChTsc*—indicates a change in *Total score* attribute (from Newman Questionnaire/Tinnitus Handicap Inventory). Second derived column-*ChTaw*—indicates a change in tinnitus awareness (*Aw T* attribute), as registered in an interview form. These changes are calculated as a difference between current value and value registered from the previous form of the given patient. Besides absolute changes, additional columns, denoting percentage changes (indicator's change related to the previous value) were developed—*PerChTsc* and *PerChTaw* (when previous value was 0, the change is 0). Next, changes were categorized, based on the frequency of change magnitude, as computed for the dataset.

8.1.4 Imputation of Missing Features

As already indicated, *Total score* attribute is missing for about half of visits registered in the tinnitus database. In other words, not every patient's visit was scored with Newman form's responses. The same applies to the second indicator—*Tinnitus awareness*. Also, when those two indicators are considered together (either *T sc* or *Aw t* value available), still, there is about 40% of the values missing. Adding further indicators does not ameliorate this situation significantly (as they are taken from the same form as *Aw t*—their availability is not greater than that of *Aw t* value).

Nevertheless, visits with no registered values of *Total score* nor *Tinnitus aware-ness* should not be omitted from the analysis. Corresponding tuples may contain treatment actions, which potentially contributed to a change, but were applied in between two scorings. Therefore, following approach was taken for imputation of missing values of score changes: each tuple of a visit that has no indicator value registered (and corresponding NULL value of a score change), is imputed with a change value from the next closest visit, when scoring was performed. It is a common-sense approach, as in this way, each potential treatment action is labeled with an effect it brings, in terms of score change. This assumption simplifies the fact that several actions might have been taken from the last to the next scoring, and the corresponding change might result from only one of such an action or, for example, of synergistic effect of all actions taken in between each total score measurement.

Imputation Algorithm Illustration

Let us consider an example of a patient, with visit history as illustrated in Table 8.1, who had only four measurements of total score *Sc t*. Therefore, only four tuples (of visits 1, 6, 7, 8) out of his 8 visits in total, would, normally, be considered in action rule extraction (half of his visits and all the information associated with them would be omitted).

The proposed approach assumes that all treatment actions performed after one total score measurement and preceding next total score measurement contribute to the registered change between the previous and the next measurements. Therefore, in the presented example, treatment actions taken at visits 2, 3, 4 and 5, whose direct effectiveness was not measured with the form, are assumed to contribute to a change in total score registered at next, 6th visit. In other words, treatment actions that took place between neighboring total score measurements (for example, between visits 1 and 6), are labeled with the change in score between these two measurements. *ChTsc* denotes absolute change in total score between two consecutive

Table 8.1 Illustration of approach to missing value imputation on a real example of patient's visits (THC = 00004)

V	Treatment action	Sc t	ChTsc	PerChTsc
0	Instr—GHS	NULL	0	0
1	Instr—GHS TRI-COE	38	0	0
2	Instr—GHS, Tel contact	NULL	−26	−68
3	Tel contact	NULL	−26	−68
4	Tel contact	NULL	−26	−68
5	Tel contact	NULL	−26	−68
6	Instr—GHH, tel contact	12	−26	−68
7	Instr—GHH, REM, audiol and counsel	18	6	50
8	Instr—GHH, REM, audiol and counsel	16	−2	−11

forms (for example, between visits 6 and 1: $12 - 38 = -26$) and *PerChTsc*—percentage change—is calculated in relation to the previous value of score (for the same visits: $[(12 - 38)/38] * 100\% = -68\%$). Negative changes denote amelioration of patient's condition, while positive changes (that is, increase in total score)—worsening. Such approach allows to retain information about effectiveness of some treatments measures, such as, in this case, instrumentation with GHS and telephone contact (after applying them, the largest improvement was observed in this patient, lowering his total score from 38 to 12).

As an effect of missing values imputation, percentage of tuples with missing *Total score* value decreases down to about 20%, and corresponding percentage for *Tinnitus awareness* attribute values—down to about 16%. Tuples that have neither change for *Total score* nor *Tinnitus awareness* account to about 14%, and therefore, will be left out from the analysis. These can be understood as visits when treatment actions were performed, but whose effect is not known in terms of registered data. For example, treatment might have been applied after initial forms, but no follow-up forms have been taken to assess its effectiveness.

8.1.5 Experimental Setup with New Attributes

Newly developed columns were read into LISp-Miner data source and defined as attributes under *Temporal* group of attributes (see Table 8.2, as continuation of Table 7.1).

They were discretized according to the magnitude of change. The discretization was performed by using *equifrequent intervals* option for the definition of change attributes. Table 8.3 depicts resulting mapping of the absolute change values to the generated equifrequent intervals, for both attributes, *ChTsc* and *ChTaw*.

Negative values indicate decrease in scores' values, thus, lower tinnitus perception. Zero value means no change and positive values worsening of tinnitus perception.

Table 8.2 Temporal attributes definition in LispMiner

Group	Att name	Attribute meaning	Type	Cat	Sample
Temporal	ChTsc	Change in *Sc T* from last value	Inter	4	Better
	ChTaw	Change in *Aw T* from last value	Inter	4	Worse
	PerChTsc	Percentage change in total score	Inter	4	The same
	PerChTaw	Percentage change in tin awareness	Inter	4	Better

Table 8.3 Category names and corresponding intervals of absolute change values for *Total score* and *Tinnitus awareness*

Category name	ChTsc	ChTaw
Much better	< − 92; −12)	< − 100; −19)
Better	< − 12; 0)	< − 19; 0)
About the same	< 0; 2)	< 0; 1)
Worse	< 2; 78)	< 1; 90)

Figures 8.3 and 8.4 show frequency distribution, correspondingly, for *Total score* and *Tinnitus awareness* change attributes.

As change attributes will be used for decision attribute, there is no need to use *succeddent flexible part*. Desirable changes are already expressed by attributes' values.

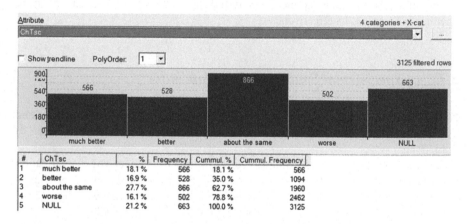

#	ChTsc	%	Frequency	Cummul. %	Cummul. Frequency
1	much better	18.1 %	566	18.1 %	566
2	better	16.9 %	528	35.0 %	1094
3	about the same	27.7 %	866	62.7 %	1960
4	worse	16.1 %	502	78.8 %	2462
5	NULL	21.2 %	663	100.0 %	3125

Fig. 8.3 Frequency distribution of total score changes' categories in tinnitus patients' visits

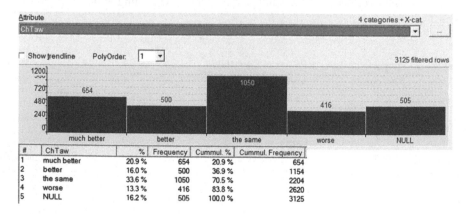

#	ChTaw	%	Frequency	Cummul. %	Cummul. Frequency
1	much better	20.9 %	654	20.9 %	654
2	better	16.0 %	500	36.9 %	1154
3	the same	33.6 %	1050	70.5 %	2204
4	worse	13.3 %	416	83.8 %	2620
5	NULL	16.2 %	505	100.0 %	3125

Fig. 8.4 Frequency distribution of categories in *ChTaw* attribute

Therefore, for the following experiments, *ChTsc* and *ChTaw* attributes (or *PerChTsc*, *PerChTaw*) were set as *succedent stable part*. Rule generation procedure checks, in this case, for which changes in flexible antecedent part, the frequency of change being "better" or "much better" increases in the given dataset.

8.2 Results

After analyzing attributes in Table 7.1 and process of treatment within TRT (Fig. 8.1), it was possible to determine stable attributes, as gender and patient's age. All other attributes are assumed to be changeable. However, if the aim of the task is to discover action rules for one particular patient, then *THC* attribute should also be set as a stable. For the purpose of other tasks' formulation, it can also be assumed that all the attributes recorded once, at the beginning of the therapy (tinnitus background, medical condition, medications taken, assigned category) are also stable, as they do not change in the course of therapy (in other words they are repeated for each visit of a given patient in the data set).

Chosen hypotheses of actions with best *Df-Conf* that lead to improvement (absolute or percentage) in either *Total score* or *Tinnitus awareness* are shown below, in groups related to one data mining task setting.

8.2.1 Treatment Protocol

Sample Ac4ft task was set up so that category assigned by doctor (*Cat*) was a stable attribute, while category chosen by a patient *CC*—flexible attribute. It is because category of treatment chosen by a doctor—assigned category—is determined at initial visit and corresponding *Cat* attribute does not change for consecutive visits for a given patient in the database. However, a patient might decide to follow a treatment protocol for the other category, and change it in the course of treatment. Therefore *CC* attribute is flexible. Succedent attributes were defined for the stable part to detect increase in relative frequency of one, positive category of change (for example, change with category "much better"). Interpretation of sample generated rule is shown below.

R:

$$Cat(1) : CC(1) \rightarrow CC(3) \implies_{0.85;158;6} ChTsc(\text{much better})$$

Initial rule:

$$Cat(1) \wedge CC(1) \implies_{F>10.148;158} ChTsc(\text{much better})$$

	ChTsc(muchbetter)	¬ChTsc(muchbetter)
Cat(1) ∧ CC(1)	158	912
¬ Cat(1) ∧ CC(1)	293	1762

$$p = \frac{158}{158+912} = 0.148, B = 158$$

Final rule:

$$Cat(1) \wedge CC(3) \implies {}_{F>11;6} \text{ChTsc(much better)}$$

	ChTsc(muchbetter)	¬ChTsc(muchbetter)
Cat(1) ∧ CC(3)	6	0
¬ Cat(1) ∧ CC(3)	445	2674

$$p = \frac{6}{6+0} = 1, B = 6$$

Interpretation

$$Cat(1) : CC(1) \rightarrow CC(3) \implies {}_{0.85;158;6} \text{ChTsc(much better)}$$
$$q = p_F - p_I = 1 - 0.148 = 0.852$$

If the treatment protocol is changed from 1 to 3 in patients diagnosed with category 1, the probability of successful treatment increases by 85% points.

Hypotheses 29 *Cat(1) : CC(1) → CC(3)* $\implies$ *$_{0.85;158;6}$ ChTsc(much better) ∧ PerChTsc(much better)*

Cat(1) : Freq LE(<2670;2800)) ∧ CC(1) → Freq LE(<3000;3150)) ∧ CC(3) $\implies$ *$_{0.89;3;3}$ ChTsc(much better) ∧ PerChTsc(much better)*

Cat(1) : FU(T) ∧ CC(1) → FU(A) ∧ CC(3) $\implies$ *$_{0.82;82;4}$ ChTsc(much better) ∧ PerChTsc(much better)*

Cat(1) : CC(0) → CC(2) $\implies$ *$_{0.36;4;4}$ ChTaw(much better)*

Cat(1) : CC(2) → CC(3) $\implies$ *$_{0.33;4;5}$ ChTaw(much better)*

Cat(1) : CC(1) → CC(2) $\implies$ *$_{0.33;4;5}$ ChTaw(much better) ∧ ChTsc(better) ∧ PerChTsc(better)*

Cat(1) : CC(1) → CC(0) $\implies$ *$_{0.079;30;3}$ ChTaw(much better) ∧ ChTsc(about the same) ∧ PerChTsc(about the same)*

8.2.2 Instrument Fitting

According to our medical expertise, in theory, all patients who do not have hyper-acusis (that is categories 0, 1, 2) can be treated without instrumentation. However, it is recommended to use some form of instrumentation to most of the patients (except category 0). One type of instruments, sound generator (SG) provides for a well-controlled, stable sound source that should lessen hyperacusis (and tinnitus) perception. Other type of instrument—hearing aid (HA) provides for additional benefit in improved hearing in patients with significant subjective hearing loss. From about 18 models of sound generators evaluated by doctor Jastreboff, he recommends to his patients most typically following devices: Viennatone, General Hearing Instrument (GHI), and sound generator from Audifon [JJ00].

The following experiment looks for desirable changes in a particular instrument fitting, that is changes in REM parameters, that can change tinnitus severity, as denoted by change in total score/tinnitus awareness category.

Hypotheses 30 *Instr(GHI):Th R SPL(< 37;38)) → Th R SPL(< 39;40))* $\Longrightarrow$ $_{0.48;5;5}$ *ChTaw(much better)*

Instr(GHI):Freq RE(< 3000;3150)) → Freq RE(< 2500;2670)) $\Longrightarrow$ $_{0.43;17;5}$ *ChTsc(much better)*

Instr(GHI):Freq RE(< 3000;3150)) → Freq RE(≥4000) $\Longrightarrow$ $_{0.34;18;6}$ *ChTsc(much better)*

Instr(GHI):Mix R SL(< 12;13)) → Mix R SL(< 4;5)) $\Longrightarrow$ $_{0.2;5;5}$ *ChTaw(much better)*

Instr(GIII):Mix R SL(< 9;10)) → Mix R SL(< 4;5)) $\Longrightarrow$ $_{0.16;6;5}$ *ChTsc(much better)*

Action rules with best confidence difference between final and initial state, were obtained for REM performed on GHI instrument. For example, the first hypothesis informs that, when threshold *Th R SPL* is increased from <37;38) to <39;40), the probability of observing changes in tinnitus awareness to be "much better" increases by 48 perc. points. The second hypothesis says that changing *Freq RE* setting from value in <3000;3150) to value in <2500;2670) increases probability of much better improvement, as indicated by total score, by 43 perc. points. Similar change of this setting to above 4000 also should increase probability of patient's condition significant amelioration (by 34 pp.). Analogous interpretation can be applied to two other action rules. Changing *GHI* instrument *Mix R SL* setting from <12;13), <9;10) to <4;5) should decrease tinnitus perception. These hypotheses should be further checked with some additional conditions on which they hold true. For example, checking for which conditions, increasing *Freq RE* from <3000;3150) improves tinnitus, and for which conditions, decreasing *Freq RE* from <3000;3150) is better.

8.2.3   Treatment Personalized for Tinnitus Induction

Following experiments in Ac4ft-Miner, with results presented below, were defined so that to obtain action rules indicating personalized treatment, taking into account individual demographic characteristics (gender and age), but also medical condition and additional diseases in a patient. They should also consider elapse of time between tinnitus/hyperacusis problem induction and treatment start, background of tinnitus induction, etc.

In the first setup, two default partial cedents were chosen for antecedent stable part: one for demographics information, and the second for boolean attributes: *M1*, *M3*, *M6*, *Y1*, *Y10*, etc. Examined actions included type of contact, instrumentation, REM, but also some demographics attributes.

Rules for Patients with Recently Induced Tinnitus (between 1–3 Months)

Hypotheses 31 $G(m) \wedge M1(yes)$: *Country(USA)* $\wedge$ *FU(A)* $\rightarrow$ *Country(Paraguay)* $\wedge$ *FU(T)* $\implies$ $_{0.79;9;6}$ *PerChTaw(much better)*

$G(m) \wedge T\,side(yes) \wedge M1(yes)$: *Country(USA)* $\wedge$ *FU(A)* $\rightarrow$ *Country(Paraguay)* $\wedge$ *FU(T)* $\implies$ $_{0.71;6;6}$ *PerChTaw(much better)*

$G(m) \wedge T\,side(yes) \wedge M1(yes)$: *Instr(HA)* $\wedge$ *Country(USA)* $\rightarrow$ *Instr(GHH)* $\wedge$ *Country(Paraguay)* $\implies$ $_{0.32;5;7}$ *PerChTaw(much better)*

$G(f) \wedge Cat(3) \wedge M1(yes)$: *FU(A)* $\rightarrow$ *FU(T)* $\implies$ $_{0.21;6;5}$ *PerChTaw(much better)*

First three rules consider male patients residing in the USA, in the "initial state of rule". Discovered knowledge quite surprisingly recommends to change country of residence to Paraguay, along with other changes, such as changing follow-up contact from "Audiological and counseling" to "Telephone", and also instrumentation treatment from "Hearing Aids" to "GH Hard". These rules were among most promising action rules found in this experiment (expected increase in "much better" change magnitude is correspondingly—79%, 71% and 32% for the first three rules). The last rule from the chosen group of hypotheses is relevant for females diagnosed with category 3, whose tinnitus started 1–3 months before therapy, and recommends changing follow-up contact from "Audiological and counseling" to "Telephone" to increase chances of relative change of tinnitus awareness to be "much better" by 21 pp.

Rules for patients with 3–12-months problem

Hypotheses 32 T $side(yes) \wedge M3(yes): Instr(GHS) \rightarrow Instr(HA) \implies_{0.7;5;8}$ $ChTaw(much\ better)$

$Cat(3) \wedge M3(yes): FU(A) \rightarrow FU(T) \implies_{0.5;5;8} PerChTsc(much\ better)$

$G(m) \wedge M6(yes): Instr(GHS) \rightarrow Instr(TCIC) \implies_{0.43;6;8} ChTsc(much\ better)$

$AgeBeg(<50;55)) \wedge M6(yes): FU(A) \rightarrow FU(T) \implies_{0.34;5;10} ChTaw(better) \wedge$ $PerChTaw(better)$

First two hypotheses consider patients, whose tinnitus started between 3 to 6 months before starting treatment, and two next—between 6 months–1 year before. First rule recommends changing instrument from "GH soft" to "Hearing aid"—then, it is expected to observe much better changes in tinnitus awareness with frequency higher by 70 pp. For category-3 patients, it recommends changing "Audiological and counseling" contact to that of "Telephone". Two next rules recommend, accordingly, changing instrumentation from instrument of "GH soft" type to "TCIC" model (which is combined instrument), and changing follow-up contact.

Rules for patients with tinnitus induced long time ago (1 year ago and before)

Hypotheses 33 $G(m) \wedge Y30(yes): FU(A) \rightarrow FU(T) \implies_{0.45;6;10} PerChTsc(better)$

$Cat(1) \wedge Y20(yes): FU(A) \rightarrow FU(T) \implies_{0.37;6;5} ChTsc(better)$

$AgeBeg(\geq 68) \wedge Y1(yes): Instr(BTE) \rightarrow Instr(GHS) \implies_{0.33;6;6} PerChTaw(much\ better)$
$G(m) \wedge Y10(yes): FU(A) \rightarrow FU(T) \implies_{0.2;13;19} PerChTaw(much\ better)$

These rules were generated for patients, whose problem started accordingly 30 years and earlier, 20–30 years ago, 1–3 years ago and 10–20 years ago. Most of them require, already well-known treatment action, of switching to "Telephone" type of contact, in order to register better change with higher probability. The third rule is valid for patients aged 68 and more, whose tinnitus started between 1–3 years ago, and recommends changing instrumentation from "BTE" model (combined instrument) to "GHS" (sound generator).

Besides time of tinnitus induction, patients should be treated individually based on the background of their tinnitus. For example, a tinnitus perception resulting from sudden exposure to noise should be approached differently than tinnitus developed gradually and associated with stressful situations in life. Examples of such action rules are presented in selected hypotheses below.

Patients with depression-induced tinnitus

Hypotheses 34   *Cat(1) $\wedge$ DETI(yes): Instr(GHS) $\rightarrow$ Instr(GHH)* $\implies$ $_{0.1;5;6}$ *PerChTsc(better)*

Above hypothesis matches patients, whose subjective perception of tinnitus onset was associated with depression, and were diagnosed with category 1 of tinnitus. It suggests, as a treatment action, switching from "GH soft" to "GH hard". Probability of change in total score to be "better" increases, then, by about 10 pp.

Patients with noise-induced tinnitus

Hypotheses 35   *G(m) $\wedge$ NTI(yes): Instr(GHS) $\wedge$ FU(T) $\rightarrow$ Instr(HA) $\wedge$ FU(A)* $\implies$ $_{0.55;5;5}$ *ChTaw(much better) $\wedge$ PerChTaw(much better)*

   G(m) $\wedge$ T side(yes) $\wedge$ NTI(yes): Occup(air traffic controller) $\rightarrow$ Occup(jazz musician) $\implies$ $_{0.47;5;6}$ *PerChTaw(better)*

   G(m) $\wedge$ NTI(yes): Instr(GHS) $\rightarrow$ Instr(Viennatone) $\implies$ $_{0.42;8;5}$ *PerChTaw(much better)*

   G(m) $\wedge$ NTI(yes): Instr(GHS) $\rightarrow$ Instr(GHH) $\implies$ $_{0.41;11;6}$ *PerChTsc(better)*

   Cat(1) $\wedge$ NTI(yes): Occup(sound engineer) $\rightarrow$ Occup(electrician) $\implies$ $_{0.3;5;5}$ *ChTaw(much better)*

   G(m) $\wedge$ T side(yes) $\wedge$ NTI(yes):Occup(air traffic controller) $\rightarrow$ Occup(pathologist) $\implies$ $_{0.32;5;7}$ *ChTsc(much better) $\wedge$ PerChTsc(much better)*

There were quite many hypotheses generated for noise-induced tinnitus patients with significant confidence difference between final and initial states, and change attributes belonging to categories "much better" or "better". Generally, recommended actions included switching from "GH soft" to other instruments ("HA", "GHH", "Viennatone"), changing telephone contact, but also, quite surprisingly, changing occupation. For example, hypotheses listed as second and the last one, recommend changing occupation from "air traffic controller" to either a "jazz musician" or "pathologist". The fifth rule's variable antecedent part is: *Occup(sound engineer)$\rightarrow$ Occup(electrician)*. The explanation, for this quite surprising change suggestion, can be that in case of tinnitus associated with exposure to noise, some occupations might be adversely affecting patient's improvement during therapy. Certainly, occupations such as air traffic controller or sound engineer are related to exposure to loud sounds, which might hinder effectiveness of the whole therapy.

Patients with stress-induced tinnitus

Hypotheses 36 $G(m) \wedge Cat(1) \wedge STI(yes): Instr(GHS) \rightarrow Instr(GHH) \implies_{0.4;5;6}$ *ChTsc(much better) / PerChTsc(much better)*

Relevant hypotheses for patients with stress-induced tinnitus, who were additionally males belonging to category 1 of tinnitus, suggests changing from "GH soft" to "GH hard", in order to register more significant improvement (absolute or percentage).

Patients with tinnitus related to some medical condition

Hypotheses 37 $G(m) \wedge Cat(1) \wedge OMTI(yes) \wedge T\,side(yes): Instr(GHS) \rightarrow Instr(GHH)$ $\implies_{0.3;10;7} PerChTaw(much\ better)$

$G(m) \wedge Cat(1) \wedge OMTI(yes) \wedge T\,side(yes): FU(T) \rightarrow FU(A) \implies_{0.062;7;8} Per$-*ChTsc(much better)*

In case of patients, whose tinnitus was registered as having background in a medical condition, recommended treatment actions also included change from "GH soft" to "GH hard", and secondly "Telephone" to "Audiology/counseling" contact (although the observable improvement is expected to be less than with the first action).

8.2.4 Treatment Personalized for Medical Condition

For the purpose of experiments considering patient's medical condition, a stable antecedent part for relevant rules was set as two partial cedents. One partial cedent involved all demographics and tinnitus-induction related attributes, and at least 2 of them had to be included in the generated pattern (minimum length of the partial cedent set to 2). The second partial cedent for stable antecedent was any attribute from *Medical condition* group set with minimum length of 1 (at least one literal had to be chosen from diseases). The flexible antecedent part was set up as conjunction of at least two attributes, understood as treatment action: instrument type and model, type of counseling, but also other changeable attributes, involving demographics: country, state of residence, work status, occupation and number of medications taken.

The most significant rules were obtained for male patients with depression disorder, arthritis, cholesterol problems, and hypertension, whose tinnitus was associated with taking medications. Possible explanation for rules considering these afflictions is that patients with them were most numerous in the population of patients. Examples of generated hypotheses along with significance values are shown below.

Patients with psychological disorders

Hypotheses 38 $G(m) \wedge T\,side(yes) \wedge Depression\,disorder(yes)$: $State(GA) \wedge FU(A)$
$\rightarrow State(WI) \wedge FU(T) \implies {}_{0.84;8;9} ChTsc(much\,better) /PerChTsc(much\,better)$

$G(m) \wedge T\,side(yes) \wedge Depression\,disorder(yes)$: $Instr(GHS) \wedge State(NY) \rightarrow$
$Instr(HA) \wedge State(WI) \implies {}_{0.45;11;8} ChTaw(much\,better)$

$G(m) \wedge T\,side(yes) \wedge seizures(yes)$: $Instr(BCIC) \wedge FU(A) \rightarrow Instr(HA) \wedge FU(T)$
$\implies {}_{0.3;8;10} ChTsc(much\,better)$

$Cat(1) \wedge T\,side(yes) \wedge Depression\,disorder(yes)$: $MedNr(\geq 5) \wedge Work(h) \rightarrow$
$MedNr(<3;4)) \wedge Work(w) \implies {}_{0.24;11;8} ChTaw(better)$

$Cat(1) \wedge T\,side(yes) \wedge Depression\,disorder(yes)$: $Instr(Viennatone) \wedge Work(h)$
$\rightarrow Instr(GHH) \wedge$

$Work(w) \implies {}_{0.22;8;9} PerChTsc(better)$

Obtained action rules are relevant for patients with depression disorder and seizures, whose tinnitus was associated with taking medicines (for these disorders). Examples of hypotheses above, show only chosen subset of the most interesting rules with the greatest promise, as for the condition's improvement. These rules are characterized by considerable *DConf* and support in both initial and final state.

Some of the hypotheses, shown above, suggest changing state of residence (for example from Georgia, New York to Wisconsin), and additionally changing either contact from "Audiological/counseling" to "Telephone" (first hypothesis) or instrumentation, from "GH soft" to "hearing aids" (second hypothesis). In case of seizures (third hypothesis) it should be beneficial to switch from "BCIC" model to "hearing aid" (the probability of success in treatment increases by 30 pp.). When treating patients from category 1 with depression disorder (hypotheses fourth and fifth), recommended actions include: changing employment status from "staying at home" to "actively working", changing sound-generator from "Viennatone" to "GH hard".

Patients with arthritis

Hypotheses 39 $G(m) \wedge T\,side(yes) \wedge arthisis(yes)$: $Instr(BTE) \wedge FU(A) \rightarrow$
$Instr(GHH) \wedge FU(T) \implies {}_{0.39;8;9} PerChTaw(much\,better)$

For male patients with arthritis, whose tinnitus is associated with medications, desirable treatment action comprises of: changing from "audiology/counseling" contact to "telephone" and instrumentation from "BTE" model to "GHH". The expected probability of treatment success increases then by almost 40 pp.

Patients with hypertension

Hypotheses 40 $G(m) \wedge T\,side(yes) \wedge cholesterol\,problems(yes) \wedge hypertension(yes)$:
$Med(\geq 5) \wedge FU(A) \rightarrow Med(<3;4)) \wedge FU(T) \implies _{0.21;19;10} PerChTaw(much\ better)$

$G(m) \wedge T\,side(yes) \wedge hypertension(yes): Instr(GHH) \wedge FU(T) \rightarrow Instr(BTE) \wedge$
$FU(A) \implies _{0.19;10;8} PerChTaw(much\ better)$

For male patients with hypertension should work either: reducing medications from
"5 and higher" to "3" and contact change from "audiological/counseling" to "telephone" (when they also have cholesterol problems) or changing from "GH hard"
sound generator to "BTE" model. It is expected that observable relative change in
tinnitus will be "much better" with, correspondingly, 21 and 19 pp. greater probability.

8.3 Meta Actions Discovery Experiment

Doctor Jastreboff states, that the main disadvantage of the Tinnitus Retraining Therapy is that the protocol has to focus on the individual needs and profile of a patient,
and consequently takes significant time of involvement of the personnel providing
the treatment, who has to be also specifically trained [JJ00]. In order to pursue greater
personalization in treatment, another approach for data mining in LISp-Miner on a
given dataset of visits and patients was proposed. The experiment was designed to
consider changes only within one course of therapy treatment (one patient's visit
history) and later, in the RS, check if the pattern is also valid for a new patient under
treatment. Therefore, analytical problem changes from finding action rules to finding
meta actions (finding set of actions for particular patients that indeed contributed to
changing tinnitus severity). After obtaining effective actions that lead to improvement
in a particular patient, characteristics of this particular patient have to be determined,
along with checking whether they are similar to a new patient under treatment. This
approach presents another way of possible mechanism to be implemented within
RECTIN system. Discovered sets of treatment actions would be fitted to a patient
profile.

8.3.1 Output

Ac4ft task within LISp-Miner was defined so that to discover meta actions, that is,
set of actions that lead to improvement (see Definition 4.6.1). The assumption is that
the actions are searched within one particular patient's visit dataset (*THC* attribute
is defined as stable). Example of generated meta actions, for particular patients in
given categories, are shown as hypotheses below:

Effective meta actions

Hypotheses 41 *THC(01053) ∧ Cat(3): CC(3) → CC(2)* $\Longrightarrow$ $_{0.67;3;3}$ *ChTsc(better)*
→ ChTsc(much better)

THC(00061) ∧ Cat(3): FU(T) → FU(A) $\Longrightarrow$ $_{0.58;3;3}$ *ChTsc(worse) →*
ChTsc(much better)

THC(99021) ∧ Cat(1): Instr(GHS) → Instr(Viennatone) $\Longrightarrow$ $_{0.56;3;3}$
ChTsc(about the same) → ChTsc(better)

THC(03085) ∧ Cat(3): CC(2) → CC(3) $\Longrightarrow$ $_{0.33;4;3}$ *ChTsc(about the same) →*
ChTsc(much better)

THC(01054) ∧ Cat(1): FU(T) → FU(A) $\Longrightarrow$ $_{0.25;3;3}$ *ChTsc(the same) →*
ChTsc(much better)

THC(03060) ∧ Cat(3): CC(2) → CC(3) $\Longrightarrow$ $_{0.17;3;4}$ *ChTsc(about the same) →*
ChTsc(much better)

THC(00045) ∧ Cat(1): Instr(GHS) → Instr(Viennatone) $\Longrightarrow$ $_{0.09;5;4}$
ChTsc(worse) → ChTsc(much better)

For some patients from category 3, it seemed to be more effective to follow treatment
protocol typical for category 2 (first hypothesis), while for the others from this category, protocol suitable for category 3 is more effective. Hypotheses fourth and sixth
say that changing treatment protocol from 3 to 2 in patients with ordering number
03085 and 03060, brings change in THI total score from better to much better, by 33
and 17 pp., correspondingly.

It is interesting to see, that although the rules were extracted for one particular
case of patient, there are more than one tuples that support initial and final state of
an action rule (BASE parameters BEFORE and AFTER were set at 3). It means that
the treatment actions were continued for at least 3 visits of a given patient. When
BASE parameter is decreased to 2, even more meta actions with higher confidence
difference, are generated for particular patients. As a matter of fact, it is possible to
extract all effective actions for each single patient (with BASE set to 1). Examples,
generated for patients in different categories, with BASE = 2, are shown below.

Effective meta actions with lower support

Hypotheses 42 *THC(00061) ∧ Cat(3): Instr(GHS) → Instr(GHH)* $\Longrightarrow$ $_{0.71;2;3}$
ChTaw(the same) → ChTaw(much better)

$THC(00022) \wedge Cat(2): FU(A) \rightarrow FU(T) \Longrightarrow_{0.64;5;2} ChTaw(worse) \rightarrow ChTaw(much\ better)$

$THC(99062) \wedge Cat(4): Instr(TCIC) \rightarrow Instr(Viennatone) \Longrightarrow_{0.5;2;4} ChTaw(worse) \rightarrow ChTaw(much\ better)$

$THC(03066) \wedge Cat(1): Freg\ LE(<3000;3150)) \rightarrow Freg\ LE(<2000;2120)) \Longrightarrow_{0.33;2;3} ChTsc(worse) \rightarrow ChTsc(about\ the\ same)$

$THC(04055) \wedge Cat(2): Instr(BTE) \rightarrow Instr(TCIC) \Longrightarrow_{0.33;2;4} ChTsc(worse) \rightarrow ChTsc(better)$

Aggravating Meta Actions

On the other hand, it is also possible to extract set of actions that are expected not to be successful. They also can be potentially implemented in the RS so that to "suggest" which actions not to take in a particular case.

Hypotheses 43 $THC(99021) \wedge Cat(1): Instr(GHS) \rightarrow Instr(GHH) \Longrightarrow_{0.56;4;3} ChTaw(much\ better) \rightarrow ChTaw(better)$

$THC(99004) \wedge Cat(2): FU(T) \rightarrow FU(A) \Longrightarrow_{0.57;3;3} ChTsc(much\ better) \rightarrow ChTsc(better)$

$THC(00052) \wedge Cat(1): Instr(GHS) \rightarrow Instr(GHH) \Longrightarrow_{0.5;3;3} ChTsc(much\ better) \rightarrow ChTsc(better)$

$THC(03068) \wedge Cat(0): CC(0) \rightarrow CC(2) \Longrightarrow_{0.4;3;4} ChTsc(better) \rightarrow ChTsc(worse)$

$THC(04032) \wedge Cat(3): CC(3) \rightarrow CC(1) \Longrightarrow_{0.3;4;4} ChTsc(better) \rightarrow ChTsc(worse)$

8.4 Discussion

8.4.1 Advantages

Experiments with the use of imputed decision attribute values of total score/tinnitus awareness changes, generated results with significant confidence difference between final and initial states. Some of them seem especially promising with an increase in treatment success by more than 80% points. Also, found rules were characterized by a considerable support, which might be contributed to the imputation of missing values.

It was possible to find relevant rules for almost each defined case of treated patient. In comparison to experiments described in the previous chapter, new interesting and potentially useful knowledge was discovered.

Also, approach to discover meta actions was proposed. Extracted sets of actions are relevant for particular patients, whose profile can serve for matching with a new case of patient under treatment. The problem, then, translates to calculating similarity measures between patients, or matching patients based on similar features, while knowing what kind of actions actually worked for a particular "class" of a patient. This approach can, potentially, be the most reliable. On the other hand, tinnitus requires such an individual treatment dependent on many factors, that even such approach does not guarantee 100% success.

8.4.2 Flaws

Action rules discovered in the above experiments provide some insight into treatment actions that have potential to improve patient's tinnitus. Actions are personalized because are detected for patients who share some features, such as age, gender, tinnitus cause, or medical condition. However, results obtained within these experiments should be taken with caution. Despite many advantages the proposed approach brings, due to some questionable assumptions made at an experimental setup, following flaws are noticed:

- change attributes are not related temporarily, that is, approach does not consider length of particular treatment action—point in time when the action was introduced and point in time when the change was observed,
- established definition of a change in score (as difference from the last measurement) labels actions, performed at a visit when first measurement was taken, as having no effect (0 value of change)—see tuple with visit 1 in Table 8.4,
- consequently, approach assumes that actions taken at a time when measurement with forms was performed, have immediate effect, reflecting their effect on forms taken at the same time—which in reality happens very rarely, taking into account time taken to habituate tinnitus,
- despite having change attributes on two indicators—*Total score* and *Tinnitus awareness*—rules are generated independently for each of the change attribute. Therefore, advantage of minimizing number of missing values with both indicators at a time is not realized.

8.4.3 Algorithm Reexamined

Let us analyze table of sample patient's visit history in Table 8.4 once again.

Table 8.4 Flaws associated with algorithm on missing values imputation

V	Treatment action	Sc t	ChTsc	PerChTsc
0	Instr—GHS	NULL	0	0
1	Instr—GHS TRI-COE	38	0	0
2	Instr—GHS, Tel contact	NULL	−26	−68
3	Tel contact	NULL	−26	−68
4	Tel contact	NULL	−26	−68
5	Tel contact	NULL	−26	−68
6	Instr—GHH, tel contact	12	−26	−68
7	Instr—GHH, REM, audiol and counsel	18	6	50
8	Instr—GHH, REM, audiol and counsel	16	−2	−11

First total score was obtained at a visit number 1, when also treatment action, in the form of instrumentation—"GHS" sound generator, was applied. This action was labeled by the algorithm as having "0" effect on tinnitus change. Nevertheless, intuitively, observing the history of actions taken, something quite opposite would be true. It seems that all that time that elapsed up to the next measurement at the 6th visit, should be considered as time of therapy with GHS instrumentation (no sooner than at the 6th visit instrumentation was changed to "GH hard"). Therefore, this action should be actually labeled as having attenuating effect on tinnitus perception.

On the other hand, we can see that at the 6th visit, when a different instrumentation was prescribed (doctor decided to switch to GH hard), this action was labeled by the algorithm as having an instant effect of decreasing tinnitus onerousness. According to medical practice, GH soft were breaking down frequently and it turned out that they could not be used. By looking at the history, we would rather conclude that this action was not effective and even increased score measuring tinnitus severity (at least with the first fitting). We can also see that while observing deterioration of patient's condition, doctor decided to take additional action of instrumentation fitting (with REM method) and also changed contact from "Telephone" to "Audiology and counseling". So, finally "GHH" with the right fitting improved patient's condition (it can be explained from medical point of view that patient finally started getting consistent and not interrupted by broken device sound stimulation). Nevertheless, at the beginning, when it was not fitted, it deteriorated tinnitus, while algorithm inadequately labeled the action as bringing "much better" change (−26).

Also, the treatment actions at the last visit were labeled as having "−2" effect, but, as a matter of fact, its effectiveness, in a time elapse was not measured (it was the last visit). It should be also asked, if labeling treatment action at visit 0, as having change of "0" is adequate. Value of "0" conveys specific information that the action taken brought no result: neither positive nor negative. However, in case of initial visits, we actually have no information of the action effect (because we have no starting value, or reference value), so we might think if "NULL" or "UNKNOWN" value would not be more suitable, for this algorithm. If yes, then probably the percentage of imputed missing values was overestimated, as the algorithm irrelevantly labeled action as "0" instead of "NULL".

Another question is, if actions taken at different points of time (and correspondingly different length of treatment), can be labeled with the same effectiveness (expressed as a change in score). Tinnitus treatment actions, as each treatment, have to take some time to bring effect. So, can we really compare an action, whose effectiveness was measured a week after its introduction, to an action with the same change value, but registered after 3 months? It can be also undermined, if a change from 38 to 12 is of the same relevance as change from 12 to 38 points of total score. Can we really use absolute change values, without relating it to previous level? Should be a percentage change used as more adequate?

To sum up, the reexamination of the algorithm brings conclusion that some assumptions on which it is based, are not acceptable, and not adequate for the dataset. Therefore, a new change attribute should be proposed, defined differently, in a manner suitable for the problem and the dataset. One final attribute is needed so that to address all the questionable assumptions discussed above, and generate final action rules for RECTIN system.

Chapter 9
Experiment 4: Treatment Rules Enhancement

Abstract Experiments on action rules, described in the previous section, did not consider temporal dependencies between patient's visits (that is, at what relative point in timeline particular actions were taken). On the other hand, it would be effective to search for temporal dependencies between particular treatment actions and their observable results in the form of changed score denoting tinnitus severity. New approach should allow to assess treatment action effectiveness in temporal terms and consider their sequence. For example, some actions might take effect after some time elapse and not be effective in the short-term.

9.1 Methodology

In order to address issues, as mentioned in discussion of the previous chapter, a new attribute, suitable for the succedent part of relevant patterns for action rule, was developed, so that to label particular treatment actions, in terms of their effectiveness, in an adequate way.

9.1.1 New Temporal Feature Development

Let us define a new change attribute for X indicator at visit v of a given patient, in a following way:

© Springer International Publishing AG 2017

K.A. Tarnowska et al., *Decision Support System for Diagnosis and Treatment of Hearing Disorders*, Studies in Computational Intelligence 685,
DOI 10.1007/978-3-319-51463-5_9

Definition 9.1 $CH_{X,v} =$

- *NULL, for* $X_n = NULL$ or $X_{n+1} = NULL$
- *0, for* $X_n = 0$ and $X_{n+1} = 0$
- $\frac{-100}{dist_{n+1,n}}$, *for* $X_n = 0$ and $X_{n+1} > 0$
- $(100\% * \frac{X_{n+1}-X_n}{X_n})/(dist_{n+1,n})$, *for* $X_n \neq 0$

where:

- $X = Tsc$ or $X = Taw$
- X_n *is measurement of* X *at* v, *or the closest previous measurement of* X *from* v: $DATE(v) \geq DATE(X_n)$
- X_{n+1} *is the closest next measurement of* X *from visit* v: $DATE(v) < DATE(X_{n+1})$
- *dist is a distance defined as below:*

Definition 9.2 $dist_{n+1,n} =$

- *NULL, for* $CH_{X_n,v} = NULL$
- *DATEDIFF*$(weeks, DATE(X_{n+1}), DATE(X_n))$, *for* $DATE(X_{n+1}) > DATE(X_n)$

Algorithm

Algorithm calculates change and distance values for each visit based on the definitions presented above:

- "change" column for a particular visit tuple, associated with some treatment actions, is generally understood as difference between next measurement of total score and measurement taken at the time of introducing the treatment action (between current *Sc T* value and next closest *Sc T* value), if, however, there is no next value to compare with, we assume that effects of the measurement cannot be assessed, and the change attribute is assigned NULL,
- for visits with treatment actions introduced at the time, when no reference measurement was taken (visit tuples without *Sc T*), the difference is calculated between closest preceding measurement and closest next measurement (between previous *Sc T* value and next closest *Sc T* value), if, however, there is either no next or no previous value to compare with, we assume that effects of the treatment measure cannot be assessed, and the corresponding change attribute is assigned NULL,
- the calculated difference is related to the current (or the previous) value of indicator—change is expressed as a percentage change (divided by current/previous value and multiplied by 100). In this way, relative changes of different indicators, such as total score or tinnitus awareness, can be compared,
- if the current/previous value is 0, we cannot divide as above: if the next value is 0, then change is 0, if the next value is greater than 0, it means than the patient's condition aggravated, and the relative difference is set to -100%.

- in order to calculate treatment action effectiveness for a time unit, the relative change is further divided by a distance, where distance is defined as a time difference in weeks between current visit date and date of the next visit when measurement was taken—this way distance informs how long the treatment action continued until it was assessed,
- the resulting change attribute is a small decimal number and expresses percentage improvement per week of treatment with a given method,
- two change and distance attributes are defined separately for two indicators: $Sc\ T$ and $Aw\ T$—resulting in 4 new features: $ChTsc$, $distTsc$, $ChTaw$, $distTaw$,
- as a result of algorithm, some tuples (visits with associated treatment) have change attributes calculated for both of these indicators ($ChTsc$ is not NULL and $ChTaw$ is not NULL), the others have change attribute just for one of these, and the rest have attribute for none of them (see example in Table 9.1). In order to take advantage from both of them combined (consider both at a time) there is a need to merge these two change features into one, final change attribute Ch and distance (length of treatment) associated with this change $distCh$.

One final change attribute

Let us define a final, combined change attribute as follows:

Definition 9.3 $CH = ChTsc$ and $distCh = distTsc$ in the following cases (in order of priority):

- Ch_{Tsc} is not *NULL* and Ch_{Taw} is *NULL*—this is the most obvious case—we choose a change in indicator that is available,
- ScT is not *NULL* and AwT is *NULL*—the case when both of change features are available for the tuple, but change for $Sc\ t$ is accurate, while $ChTaw$ is approximated by "neighboring" previous and next measurements,
- Ch_{Tsc} is not *NULL* and Ch_{Taw} is not *NULL* and $distTsc < distTaw$—there are values for change attributes for both indicators, as well as current values of indicators themselves ($Sc\ t$ and $Aw\ T$)—a change value associated with lower distance is chosen (it is assumed that treatment effectiveness measured in shorter time distance is more accurate).

Analogously:

$CH = ChTaw$ and $distCh = distTaw$

when:

- Ch_{Tsc} is *NULL* and Ch_{Taw} is not *NULL*,
- ScT is *NULL* and AwT is not *NULL*
- Ch_{Tsc} is not *NULL* and Ch_{Taw} is not *NULL* and $distTsc > distTaw$.

The last case, not resolved by the two above, is when Ch_{Tsc} is not *NULL* and Ch_{Taw} is not *NULL* and $distTsc = distTaw$. Then a "combined" change is calculated as an average of both:

Table 9.1 Illustration of algorithm determining Ch and $distCh$ on a chosen example of patient with ordering number (THC) 04014

V	Treatment action(s)	Date	Sc t	Aw t	Ch_{Tsc}	Ch_{Taw}	d_{Tsc}	d_{Taw}	Ch	dCh
0	Aud, TRICOE, FU(A)	2004-02-09	N	20	N	0	N	8	**0**	**8**
1	CO, TCIC, FU(A)	2004-02-23	N	N	N	0	N	6	**0**	**6**
2	TCIC, FU(A)	2004-04-05	0	20	0	−11	7	7	**−5**	**7**
3	TCIC, REM, FU(A)	2004-05-24	0	5	−5	0	22	8	**0**	**8**
4	TCIC, FU(T)	2004-07-22	N	5	−7	9	14	7	**9**	**7**
5	TCIC, REM, FU(A)	2004-09-07	N	8	−14	21	7	7	**21**	**7**
5	TCIC, REM, FU(A)	2004-09-07	N	8	−14	21	7	7	**21**	**7**
6	TCIC, FU(T)	2004-10-27	2	20	0	−2	6	28	**0**	**6**
7	Aud, HA, REM, FU(A)	2004-12-07	2	N	−8	−3	12	22	**−8**	**12**
8	TCIC, REM, FU(A)	2005-03-02	0	N	0	−6	10	10	**0**	**10**
9	TCIC	2005-05-10	0	8	N	N	N	N	**N**	**N**

$$CH = \frac{Ch_{Tsc}+Ch_{Taw}}{2} \text{ and } distCh = distTaw = distTsc.$$

Algorithm illustration

Let us track the algorithm of feature development and imputation on the real example of a single patients' visit history (with THC = 04014), as presented in Table 9.1.

Patient with THC = 04014 (that is, 14th registered patient in year '04) has 10 visits registered. Visit 5 has two tuples, as there were two different instrument fittings (REM) at the same day. It can be seen that for some of his/her visits, a measurement of $Sc\ t$ (total score from Neumann form) is missing. On the other hand, there is quite a good inventory of tinnitus awareness measurements $Aw\ t$ (taken from initial/follow-up interview forms). Treatment actions undertaken for this patient include instrumentation, REM fitting and counseling. It can be noticed that throughout the therapy, treatment was changing, in terms of different types of instruments, subsequent fittings, and follow-up contacts (audiology/counseling, telephone). For example, at visit 1, doctor changed instrumentation from sound generator of "TRI-COE" model to combined instrument of "TCIC" model. He changed instrumentation at visit 7 once again (to "HA"—hearing aid), but returned to combined instrument ("TCIC") at visit 8. At visits 4 and 6, doctor switched contact from "Audiology/counseling" to "Telephone", and reverse changes were introduced at visits 5 and 7.

Presented in the table $ChTsc$, $ChTaw$, $dTsc$, $dTaw$ columns are derived attributes, calculated by algorithm based on definitions presented in the previous sections. Although they are calculated and stored in the database as 4 digit-scale decimals, the table shows calculated values of $ChTsc$ and $ChTaw$ as integers, to simplify an example. Distance is calculated as time difference between current visit date and date of the next visit when measurement was taken (they express length of treatment that is measurable in terms of effectiveness). Based on these four additional attributes and established definitions, a final change attribute—Ch, with corresponding distance dCh—is determined (bold values in the table). It can be noticed that finally only one value for Ch is missing.

Detailed tracking of measures taken and their corresponding effects as changes in $Sc\ t$ and $Aw\ t$, helps to drive some conclusions. For example, treatment actions taken at visit 0 and 1, brought no effect ($Aw\ t$ of the next visit—2, has not changed in relation to the previous value). Change $ChTaw$ for treatment undertaken at visit 0 is calculated as $100\% * \frac{20-20}{20}/8 = 0$, and the same way for visit 1 (as there was no Aw t for this visit, for difference calculation the closest previous value was taken—20 from visit 0). As for these two visits, we do not know effects, in terms of total score (there are no corresponding $ChTsc$ values), the final change for Ch is taken from $ChTaw$ attribute.

For the visit 2 we have current values for both total score and tinnitus awareness. $ChTsc$ for visit 2 is 0, as the current and the next value of $Sc\ t$ are 0. $ChTaw$ is calculated as: $100\% * \frac{5-20}{20}/7 = -10,7142\%$. As distances for $dTsc$ and $dTaw$ are equal (both are 7 weeks), the final change attribute is calculated as an average between $ChTsc$ and $ChTaw$: $Ch = 100\% * \frac{0+(-10,7142)}{2} = -5$.

$ChTsc$ for visits 4 and 5 can be calculated based on $Sc\ t$ from visits 3 and 6. The change is from 0 to 2 and, according to the definition established (and based on the fact that we cannot divide by 0 - which happens to be the previous value in this case), is calculated as $100\%/dTsc$, which equals to $100\%/14$ and $100\%/7$ correspondingly for the 4th and 5th visit. $ChTaw$ for these visits is calculated with the use of standard equation for a change in values from 5 to 8, and from 8 to 20. In both cases the tinnitus awareness increased, that is patient's condition worsened. It is expressed by corresponding 9 and 21 values of $ChTaw$ for visits 4 and 5. It can also be observed that according to $ChTsc$ value, treatment undertaken at visits 4 and 5 was effective, while according to $ChTaw$—worsened tinnitus. Algorithm decides which values are more reliable—as $Aw\ t$ was taken directly at the time of introducing the treatment and directly at the next visit, while $Sc\ t$ was taken some time before the treatment and was measured only after some other treatment was applied—more reliable measure for change would be $ChTaw$ (according to the definition, this attribute is chosen for Ch, because $Sc\ t$ for these visits are NULL).

For visit 6 there is a reverse situation: $ChTsc$ is calculated directly between the current and the very next value, while $ChTaw$ was approximated, as difference between current measure and the one taken three visits later (at visit 9). Therefore according to the analogous assumption, the final Ch and dCh are taken as $ChTsc$ and $dTsc$ values. The same logic is relevant to visit 7, with $ChTsc$ calculated as $100\% * \frac{0-2}{2}/12 = -8,3333\%$, and to visit 8 (with change from 0 to 0 defined as

0). For the last visits we can never calculate effectiveness of treatment actions introduced at them, as there are no corresponding "next" values. But, looking at the sample history of a patient's visit, some labels assessing effectiveness of treatment with TCIC instrument were developed. As a matter of fact, most visits for this patient included treatment with this model of combined instrumentation.

Concluding this example, there are some treatment actions labeled as having no effect ($Ch = 0$), for example, instrumentation treatment with "TRICOE", some that have positive effect (instrumentation with "HA", instrument fitting, counseling) and most of visit's actions are labeled as deteriorating patient's condition (by 6–12%)— for example, treatment with "TCIC" and its fitting proved not very successful.

9.1.2 Experimental Setup

A new attribute Ch (with corresponding $distCh$ attribute) was introduced to LISp-Miner environment under *Temporal* group of attributes (see Table 9.2).

Figure 9.1 shows categories defined for Ch attribute, as intervals, along with their balanced frequency (absolute, relative and cumulated).

There are 5 categories for change value: "worse" for positive values of Ch, "about the same" for no change, and three categories for different magnitudes of negative

Table 9.2 Ch and *treat len* attributes definition in LISp-Miner

Group	Att Name	Attribute meaning	Type	Cat	Sample
Temporal	Ch	Percentage change per week	Inter	5	Better
	$treat_{len}$	Length of treatment in weeks	Inter	10	<1;4)

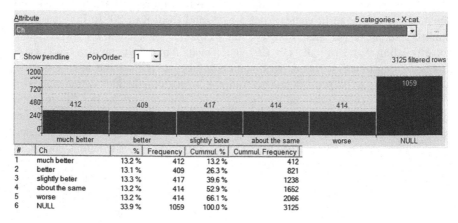

Fig. 9.1 *Frequency distribution of Ch attribute categories in tinnitus visits' dataset*

values: "slightly better", "better" and "much better". Corresponding values intervals for each category are shown in Table 9.3.

Distance features

Additional column, indicating length of treatment of a given measure (*distCh*), was defined as an interval attribute—*treat len*. In order to relate particular patient's visits temporally, following columns were also developed:

- *distPrev*—time difference (in weeks) between a given and the previous visit of the patient (for initial visit the distance is 0),
- *dist0*—for each visit: time elapse (in weeks) from initial visit, the last visit's *dist0* informs about total time of a patient's treatment,

Task setting

After additional attributes' definition in LISp-Miner, they were used for defining relevant patterns in Ac4ft tasks. Succedent part was set as disjunction of three literals: *Ch(slightly better)*, *Ch(better)*, *Ch(much better)*. Therefore, each treatment action increasing probability of improvement (no matter of the magnitude of the improvement), was taken into account. It is assumed that actions that generally lead to "better" condition are interesting (for now, no matter if improvement is slight, moderate or significant). Therefore, it is possible to obtain rules with succedent, as following disjunction: $Ch(better) \vee Ch(muchbetter) \vee Ch(slightlybetter)$. The procedure is enforced to generate only interesting action rules (from treatment point of view) and recommend only effective treatment actions, under conditions specified by stable antecedent literals.

Antecedent part definition was similar as in experiments described in the previous chapter, with one exception: when the goal of the task was to find changes in treatment length leading to improvement, treatment measures (such as instrumentation, fitting, contact) were defined in stable antecedent part. It is because, for such a scenario, the goal is to find changes of treatment length for a given method of treatment, set as fixed in this case.

Table 9.3 Category names and corresponding intervals for *Ch* attribute

Category name	Ch
Much better	$<-99; -4.9107)$
Better	$<-4.9107; -2)$
Slightly better	$<-2; 0, 4348)$
About the same	$<-0.4348; 0.8418)$
Worse	$<0.8418; 1944.7369)$

9.2   Results

With a new, accurate change attribute *Ch* for succedent part, developed as described
above, final choice of the most reliable rules for RECTIN *Rule Engine* can be made.
Generated results were obtained faster in relation to experiments described in the
previous chapters, as succedent part of relevant rule consisted of one cedent (defined
as *disjunction* of three literals, each defined as "One category" coefficient of *Ch*-
"slightly better", "better" or "much better").

Besides considering *Ch* attribute in the experimental setup, also temporal dependencies between actions and their effects were considered, suggesting changing
length of treatment with a particular method (*treat* attribute).

9.2.1   Instrument Fitting

Hypotheses 44 *Instr(GHI):Freq LE(<3000; 3150))* → *Freq LE ≥ 3775)* ⟹
$_{0.32;37;8}$ *Ch(better/much better/slightly better)*

Instr(SG): Mix R SL(<9; 10)) → *Mix R SL(<11; 12))* ⟹ $_{0.27;8;11}$ *Ch(better/
much better/slightly better)*

Instr(SG): Mix R SL(<9; 10)) → *Mix R SL(<15; 17))* ⟹ $_{0.27;8;8}$ *Ch(better/
much better/slightly better)*

Instr(GHI): Mix L SL(<7; 8)) →*Mix L SL<2* ⟹ $_{0.27;8;8}$ *Ch(better/much
better/slightly better)*

Instr(GHI): Mix L SL(<7; 8)) → *Mix L SL(<11; 12))* ⟹ $_{0.27;8;8}$ *Ch(better/
much better/slightly better)*

*Instr(SG): FreqLE(<2670; 2800)) ∧ FreqRE(<2670; 2800))→ FreqLE(<2500;
2670)) ∧ FreqRE(<2500; 2670))* ⟹ $_{0.23;6;7}$ *Ch(better/much better/slightly better)*

Instr(GHI): Th L SPL(<36; 37)) → *Th L SPL(<37; 38))* ⟹ $_{0.17;8;9}$ *Ch(better/
much better/slightly better)*

Instr(GHI): Mix R SL(<6; 7))→ Mix R SL(<9; 10)) ⟹ $_{0.17;9;8}$ *Ch(better/much
better/slightly better)*

Instr(SG): Freq RE(<3000; 3150)) → *Freq RE(<2500; 2670))* ⟹ $_{0.11;9;12}$
Ch(better/much better)

Instr(SG): Freq RE(<3000; 3150)) → *Freq RE(<2500; 2670))* ⟹ 0.03;5;6 *Ch(slightly better)* → *Ch(better/much better)*

Instr(SG): Freq LE(<2670; 2800)) → *Freq LE(<2500; 2670))* ⟹ 0.1;12;9 *Ch(better/much better/slightly better)*

Instr(SG): Freq LE(<2670; 2800)) → *Freq LE(<3000; 3150))* ⟹ 0.1;8;11 *Ch(better/much better)*

Instr(SG) ∧ Model(TR COE): Freq RE(<2500; 2670)) → *Freq RE(<2670; 2800))* ⟹ 0.09;10;10 *Ch(better/much better/slightly better)*

Instr(SG) ∧ Model(TR COE): Freq RE(<2500; 2670)) → *Freq RE(<3000; 3150))* ⟹ 0.08;10;12 *Ch(better/much better/slightly better)*

Instr(SG): Freq RE(<2670; 2800)) → *Freq RE(<2500; 2670))* ⟹ 0.08;11;12 *Ch(better/much better/slightly better)*

Instr(GHS): Freq RE(<2800; 3000)) → *Freq RE(<2670; 2800))* ⟹ 0.07;11;12 *Ch(better/much better/slightly better)*

Instr(SG): Th R SPL(<33; 34)) → *Th R SPL(<36; 37))* ⟹ 0.02;8;9 *Ch(better/ much better/slightly better)*

Type(GHH): Freq RE(<2670; 2800)) → *Freq RE(<3000; 3150))* ⟹ 0.02;8;13 *Ch(better/much better/slightly better)*

FU(A) ∧ Instr(GHI) ∧ Freq RE(<3000; 3150)): treat(<6; 8)) → *treat(<5; 6))* ⟹ 0.1;9;8 *Ch(better/much better/slightly better)*

Above action rules, related to instruments fitting with REM, include rules for the following type of instruments: "SG" (sound generators generally), "GHI" (general type of sound generator that includes both GHI hard and GHI soft models), particular types: "GHS" (GHI soft) and "GHH" (GHI hard), up to specific model, such as "TRI-COE". Therefore, these results on REM action rules, provide better insight, in comparison to the previous experimental setup, for which relevant rules were obtained only for "GHI" instrument fitting (compare with Hypotheses 30). Following settings of the instruments were considered in variable antecedent parts of rules: *Freq RE, Freq LE, Mix R SL, Mix L SL, Th R SPL, Th L SPL*. These constitute quite a significant subset of settings for instrumentation fitting. Some of the obtained results confirmed action rules from the previous experimental setup, but some of them provide a new insight into effective treatment actions.

As it was already explained, in the previous chapter, how to interpret action rules, interpretation of the single action rule from above will be omitted. In this chapter, focus will be set on action rules that suggest change in length of treatment of a particular method. For example, the last action rule from Hypotheses 44 informs that probability of successful treatment increases by 10% points, when the "Audiological/counseling" treatment combined with "GHI" instrumentation with setting of *Freq RE* in <3000; 3150) shortens from 6–8 weeks to 5–6 weeks.

9.2.2 Treatment Protocol

Action rules, related to the change of treatment protocol, as presented below, are more diverse, than corresponding Hypotheses 29 (which were discovered only for category-1 patients). The second rule from the below listing informs, for example, that changing treatment of category-0 patient from treatment protocol "0" lasting 12–16 weeks to treatment protocol "1" for more than 32 weeks, should increase improvement by 61 pp.

Hypotheses 45 *Cat(0): CC(0) → CC(1)* $\implies$ $_{0.33;42;9}$ *Ch(better/slightly better)*

Cat(0): CC(0) ∧ treat(<12; 16)) → CC(1) ∧ treat ≥ 32 $\implies$ $_{0.61;42;9}$ *Ch(better/ slightly better)*

Cat(3): Instr(GHH) ∧ FU(T) ∧ CC(3) → Instr(TCI-C) ∧ FU(A) ∧ CC(2) $\implies$ $_{0.33;8;9}$ *Ch(better/much better/slightly better)*

Cat(3): Instr(Viennatone) ∧ CC(3) → Instr(TCI-C) ∧ CC(2) $\implies$ $_{0.25;8;8}$ *Ch(slightly better/better/much better)*

Cat(3): CC(0) → CC(2) $\implies$ $_{0.18;8;22}$ *Ch(slightly better/better/much better)*

Cat(1): CC(0) → CC(1) $\implies$ $_{0.14;9;491}$ *Ch(slightly better/better/much better)*

Cat(3): CC(0) → CC(3) $\implies$ $_{0.08;8;239}$ *Ch(slightly better/better/much better)*

9.2.3 Treatment Personalized for Demographics

The following hypotheses were generated for the tasks defined so that to maximize treatment personalization. For the antecedent part, four groups of partials cedents were defined:

- demographics attributes (age, gender, occupation, work status),
- problem induction background (noise, stress, auto-accident, operation, medical, depression),
- relative time of induction (W2, M1, M3, M6, Y3, Y5, Y10, Y20, Y30),
- category of tinnitus diagnosed by a doctor.

Each of these partial cedents was defined with a minimum length of 1 (that is at least one attribute from each group had to be included in rule's antecedent literals).

Hypotheses 46 *AgeBeg(<50; 55))∧ G(m) ∧ Cat(1) ∧ T side(yes): MedNr ≥ 5 → MedNr(<2; 3))* $\implies$ $_{0.55;14;8}$ *Ch(slightly better/better)*

G(m) ∧ Cat(1) ∧ OMTI(yes) ∧ T side(yes): MedNr(<3; 4)) → MedNr(<4; 5)) $\implies$ $_{0.41;9;18}$ *Ch(slightly better/better/much better)*

AgeBeg(<50; 55))∧ G(m) ∧ AgeInd(<50; 56)) ∧ T side(yes): CC(2) → CC(1) $\implies$ $_{0.55;14;11}$ *Ch(slightly better/better/ much better)*

G(m) ∧ Cat(1) ∧ OMTI(yes) ∧ T side(yes): F(T) → F(A) $\implies$ $_{0.23;9;16}$ *Ch(slightly better/much better)*

AgeBeg(<55; 60))∧ G(m) ∧ Cat(1) ∧ T side(yes): Instr(GHS) → Instr(GHH) $\implies$ $_{0.19;8;8}$ *Ch(better/much better)*

9.2.4 Treatment Personalized for Tinnitus Background

Hypotheses 47 *OMTI(yes) ∧ T side(yes): Instr(Viennatone) ∧ FU(T) → Instr(GHH) ∧ FU(A)* $\implies$ $_{0.56;8;8}$ *Ch(slightly better/better)*

NTI(yes) ∧ G(m): Instr(GHS) → Instr(GHH) $\implies$ $_{0.33;28;8}$ *Ch(slightly better/better/much better)*

G(m) ∧ OMTI(yes) ∧ M6(yes) ∧ Cat(1): FU(T) → FU(A) $\implies$ $_{0.3;5;10}$ *Ch(slightly better/better/much better)*

OMTI(yes) ∧ T side(yes): Work(h) → Work(w) $\implies$ $_{0.3;13;11}$ *Ch(slightly better/better)*

OMTI(yes) ∧ G(f): Instr(GHS) → Instr(GHH) $\implies$ $_{0.28;10;8}$ *Ch(slightly better/better)*

OMTI(yes) ∧ T side(yes) ∧ Cat(1): Instr(GHS) → Instr(GHH) $\implies$ $_{0.3;13;11}$ *Ch(slightly better/better)*

OMTI(yes) ∧ G(f): Instr(Viennatone) → Instr(GHH) $\implies$ $_{0.25;8;8}$ *Ch(slightly better/better/much better)*

OMTI(yes) ∧ *T side(yes)* ∧ *Cat(1): Instr(Viennatone)* ∧ *FU(T)* → *Instr(GHS)* ∧ *FU(A)* ⟹ $_{0.24;8;8}$ *Ch(slightly better/better)*

G(m) ∧ *NTI(yes)* ∧ *M3(yes)* ∧ *Cat(3): FU(A)* → *FU(T)* ⟹ $_{0.18;6;8}$ *Ch(slightly better/better/much better)*

OMTI(yes) ∧ *Instr(GHS): treat≥32* → *treat(<5; 6))* ⟹ $_{0.06;9;6}$ *Ch(slightly better/better/much better)*

OMTI(yes) ∧ *FU(T): treat(<21; 32))* → *treat(<8; 10))* ⟹ $_{0.01;11;14}$ *Ch(slightly better/better/much better)*

The two last rules hypothesize that in case of medical-induced tinnitus (*OMTI(yes)*), it should be advantageous to shorten treatment with "GHS" instrumentation from "above 32 weeks" to 5–6 weeks, as well as shorten telephone treatment from 21–32 weeks to 8–10 weeks.

9.2.5   Treatment Personalized for Medical Condition

Relevant action rules, which consider other diseases in a patient, include: patient with ulcers, hypertension, seizures, depression/anxiety disorders, and treatment actions, such as: reducing number of medications (which are also associated with tinnitus as a side-effect), changing instrumentation (for example from "GHS" to "HA", or from "Viennatone" to "GHS"), but also changing place of residence (for example, state "NY" to "WI", "A" to "IL").

Hypotheses 48 *G(m)* ∧ *T side(yes)* ∧ *Ulcers(yes): Med(≥5)* ∧ *State(GA)* → *Med(<2; 3))*∧ *State(IL)* ⟹ $_{0.73;10;8}$ *Ch(slightly better/better)*

G(m) ∧ *T side(yes)* ∧ *Ulcers(yes)* ∧ *Erosive arthritis(yes)* ∧ *GERD(yes): Med(≥5)* ∧ *State(GA)* → *Med(<2; 3))*∧ *State(IL)* ⟹ $_{0.71;10;8}$ *Ch(slightly better/better)*

Cat(1) ∧ *T side(yes)* ∧ *Hypertension(yes): Med(≥5)* ∧ *FU(T)* → *Med(<4; 5))* ∧ *FU(A)* ⟹ $_{0.56;12;11}$ *Ch(slightly better/better/much better)*

G(m) ∧ *T side(yes)* ∧ *Seizures(yes): Instr(GHS)* ∧ *State(NY)* → *Instr(HA)* ∧ *State(WI)* ⟹ $_{0.53;9;8}$ *Ch(slightly better/much better)*

G(m) ∧ *T side(yes)* ∧ *Depression(yes)* ∧ *Panic disorder (yes)* ∧ *Seizures(yes): Instr(GHS)* ∧ *State(NY)* → *Instr(HA)* ∧ *State(WI)* ⟹ $_{0.53;9;8}$ *Ch(slightly better/much better)*

Cat(1) ∧ *T side(yes)* ∧ *Depression(yes)* ∧ *Anxiety disorder (yes): Instr(GHH)* ∧ *Med(≥5)* → *Instr(GHS)* ∧ *Med(<4; 5))* ⟹ $_{0.48;9;12}$ *Ch(slightly better/better/ much better)*

G(m) ∧ *T side(yes)* ∧ *Depression(yes): Med(≥5)* ∧ *State(GA)* → *Med(<2; 3)))* ∧ *State(WI)* ⟹ $_{0.47;14;10}$ *Ch(slightly better/much better)*

G(m) ∧ *T side(yes)* ∧ *Seizures(yes): Med(≥5)* ∧ *FU(A)* → *Med(<2; 3))* ∧ *FU(T)* ⟹ $_{0.47;9;8}$ *Ch(slightly better/better/much better)*

OMTI(yes) ∧ *T side(yes)* ∧ *Depression(yes): Instr(Viennatone)* ∧ *Med(≥5)* → *Instr(GHS)* ∧ *Med(<4; 5))* ⟹ $_{0.42;21;12}$ *Ch(slightly better/much better)*

9.2.6 Meta Actions

Following hypotheses show examples of meta actions generated for patient 01054 (that is, set of effective actions, for this particular patient).

Hypotheses 49 *THC(01054)* ∧ *Cat(1): Instr(VSS)* ∧ *F(T)* → *Instr(V-AMTI)* ∧ *F(A)* ⟹ $_{0.67;1;4}$ *Ch(slightly better/better/much better)*

THC(01054) ∧ *Cat(1): Freg LE(<2500; 2670))* ∧ *Freg RE(<2500; 2670))* ∧ *Mix R SPL(<51; 52))* → *Freg LE(<2120; 2380))* ∧ *Freg RE(<2380; 2500))* ∧ *Mix R SPL(<53; 55))* ⟹ $_{0.5;1;1}$ *Ch(better/much better)*

THC(01054) ∧ *Cat(1): Freg LE(<3000; 3150))* ∧ *Freg RE(<3000; 3150))* ∧ *Mix R SL(<9; 10))* → *Freg LE(<2500; 2670))* ∧ *Freg RE(<2500; 2670))* ∧ *Mix R SL(<14; 15))* ⟹ $_{0.5;1;1}$ *Ch(slightly better/much better)*

THC(01054) ∧ *Cat(1): Freg LE(<3000; 3150))* ∧ *Freg RE(<3000; 3150))* ∧ *Mix R SL(<9; 10))* → *Freg LE(<2120; 2380))* ∧ *Freg RE(<2380; 2500))* ∧ *Mix R SL(<11; 12))* ⟹ $_{0.5;1;1}$ *Ch(slightly better/better/much better)*

THC(01054) ∧ *Cat(1): Mix R SL(<13; 14))* ∧ *Mix R SPL(<51; 52))* ∧ *Th R SPL(<38; 39))* → *Mix R SL(<11; 12))* ∧ *Mix R SPL(<53; 54))* ∧ *Th R SPL(<42; 43))* ⟹ $_{0;1;1}$ *Ch(better/much better)*

The above set of actions for this particular patient (meta-actions) are examples of effective treatment undertaken for this case (profile) of a patient. It can be also observed that the last set of actions (last hypothesis) brought no effect.

9.3 Summary of Experiments on Rules Extraction

Experiments described in three previous chapters were conducted in order to extract knowledge on tinnitus diagnosis and treatment, in the form of rules—decision rules and action rules, whose theoretical background was presented in Chap. 4. While the former should help to understand relations between different diagnosis factors, the latter suggest a course of treatment action leading to improvement of a patient's condition. Experiments on finding association rules can also help in analyzing the collected data in terms of patient's characteristics and discover patterns that are not obvious from medical point of view.

However, the main advantage of the proposed approach based on rule extraction, is a possibility to automatically retrieve knowledge in the form of rules, without a medical expert engagement. It seems promising, as experts are usually not widely available and knowledge engineering based on interviewing experts is quite time-consuming. Often, it is also cumbersome for experts to formulate their knowledge in the form of specific rules, as they often make decisions intuitively, based on experience heuristics. This knowledge is, on the other hand, hidden in the database in the form of large sets of data, which can be mined for rules that imitate human behavior. This methodology is particularly interesting and useful for building a rule-based recommender system.

The discovered rules can be either exploited in a qualitative way by an expert, or used to perform classification (scoring) of incoming objects. Ultimately, automatically extracted rules should be built into the *Rule Module* of RECTIN system (see Fig. 5.2). Proper mechanism of automatic rule execution (or alternatively inference engine) should be implemented. Relevant rules could be then evoked with new patient data matching rules' premises and their outcome (conclusions) could be presented to the RECTIN system user.

One of the problem in discovering knowledge on treatment actions is quite limited information on the details of treatment provided by doctor. In particular, important information on type of counseling (or what the counseling consisted of), provided to the patients is missing. On the other hand, counseling, besides instrumentation, is vital for Tinnitus Retraining Therapy. Although there are descriptive columns with comments that can potentially provide some insight, they are sporadically entered in the database and written in shortcuts, which sometimes seem difficult to entangle for a medical novice.

Another problem of automatic rule extraction is that in case of large number of generated rules, it is difficult to assure that obtained rules are not contradictory (that is, the same antecedents lead to different, contradictory succedents). Therefore some automatic mechanism for *truth maintenance system* should be applied in RECTIN, as well. LISp-Miner experiments proved to result in many similar rules (in terms of literals selected for antecedent part, but different variations and combinations of them). Therefore, although there was generally a large number of them generated at an experiment, many of the subsequent hypotheses did not provide additional knowledge content. Also, at each experiment, different settings on antecedents' attributes and quantifiers should be adjusted.

Rule extraction, in contrary to classifier construction method, as described in Chap. 6, provides better insight into different diagnosis and treatment factors and allows customization of associations, which are aimed to be discovered. Also, when implemented into RECTIN, they can potentially provide *explanatory mechanism*. It means, decision the system arrives at, can be explained by means of rules' antecedent parts, that were matched. It can also potentially provide educational facility, as the untrained, in tinnitus treatment, personnel can learn tinnitus diagnosis and treatment using the system and its explanatory facilities, which imitate human expert behavior and decisions.

The main obstacle preventing from detecting diagnostic/treatment action rules with high confidence and support was the problem of missing attributes, which could help assess change of tinnitus perception and patient's condition. Some approximating approaches have been proposed so that to impute missing values with a sensible approach—therefore, retaining as much information as possible from a given data content.

To sum up experiments, discovered rules confronted with expert knowledge can confirm the correctness of the approach and methodology, while new unknown patterns provide additional knowledge to the expert he could not easily see in a large and complex dataset. It is important to note that the discovered knowledge should be treated as hypotheses, which nevertheless, have to be either confirmed by an expert or by a controlled study, designed to validate the hypothetical claims. In particular, rules generated and presented in this work should not be basis for any diagnosis or treatment decision, or suggest any particular course of treatment, as this work is purely experimental and aimed at showing possible application of action rules and meta action in medicine. Final check of the validity of approach can be obtained by comparison with clinical results and knowledge.

Chapter 10
RECTIN Implementation

Abstract This chapter describes prototype RECTIN implementation with regard to each component. For classification module and rule engine module, the most interesting code parts are listed.

10.1 Application

Diagram in Fig. 10.1 depicts application architecture in general environment of RECTIN system. Two yellow areas denote: analytics part (left) and transactional part (right).

Application consists of forms for patient and visit data entry, as well as for filling in the electronic forms: Initial/Follow-up Interview form and Tinnitus Handicap Inventory form. The system user should also be able to generate reports: on patient category prediction, with relevant metrics (such as accuracy), and second, on treatment action recommendation with detailed explanation section (based on matched rules). These two reports are generated by, accordingly, *Classification Component* and *Rule Engine Component*. The data is stored in the central database, whose structure will be described in the next section. It registers transactions from application. Based on the data, suitable predictions/rules are executed and results are presented in reports. Database also serves for relearning models for classification and rule extraction. Accordingly defined ETL jobs should periodically extract data from database, transform it properly for data mining tasks, and load into files, on which data mining/machine learning tasks can be performed. After "relearning" the models, the recommender facility is improved with new data.

K.A. Tarnowska et al., *Decision Support System for Diagnosis and Treatment of Hearing Disorders*, Studies in Computational Intelligence 685, DOI 10.1007/978-3-319-51463-5_10

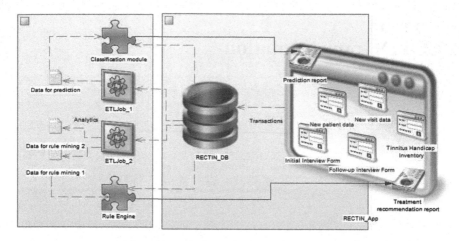

Fig. 10.1 RECTIN Application architecture diagram

10.2 Transactional Database

The original database was redesigned, so that to improve transaction efficiency, ensure data consistency, eliminate redundant data and relate data with keys. Resulting model of transactional database for RECTIN system is shown in Fig. 10.2.

In comparison to original data structure (see diagram in Fig. 5.3), data related to patients and visits was normalized (3NF) to ensure that no redundant data is stored, and enable at the same time quick retrieval of related data with simple queries (based on foreign keys). Reference tables were developed to avoid misspellings with manual data entry and ensure integrity of data, and once again—avoid repeating data. Reference tables, sometimes called "Dictionaries" should be provided with the system (the reference data should be uploaded before the use of system). Some values are expected to be automatically inserted, for example, calculation of scores in *THI* table. Additional *Counseling* table was developed so that to store details about counseling sessions, which are often missing or entered in textual form, inappropriate for knowledge discovery, but on the other hand can provide important source of information from data and rule mining point of view.

The central table is *Visit*, which can be joined with any tables storing details of treatment actions undertaken at the visit: *Instrumentation, REM, Counseling*, or any medical evaluation performed at it (*Audiological, Pharmacology*). Last but not least, the given visit can be associated with forms for tracking treatment progress: *THI* (Tinnitus Handicap Inventory, also called Newman Form), *Interview*. The latter stores all other information a physician could include when conducting personal interview. There are two views based on this table: *Initial interview* and *Follow up interview*, which should serve for developing suitable forms in the RECTIN interface.

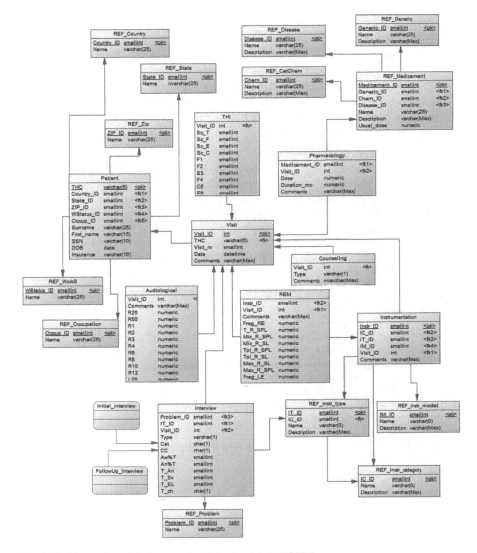

Fig. 10.2 Physical model of transactional database for RECTIN

10.3   Classification Module

Prototype classification module of RECTIN system, implemented in Java, with WEKA API is shown in Listing 10.1. The module consists of two most important functions: *learn()* and *predict()*. The former constructs the classification model, the latter performs classification on new data with built and dumped model. Themodule uses WEKA API for classification and feature selection algorithms. Example listed uses *Bayes* package with *NaiveBayes* algorithm and attribute selection based on *ChiSquaredAttributeEval*. Dataset, on which classifier is built, is retrieved from .csv file, which is periodically refreshed by ETL jobs (retrieving up-to-date data from central database—see application architecture in Fig. 10.1). The classifier is implemented as *FilteredClassifier*, that is, built with the use of filter on attributes. *Filter* is an *AttributeSelection* object, which uses *ChiSquared* attribute evaluator with *Ranker* method. The built model is dumped on disc, and used for performing prediction with new data (model is dumped with *saveModel()* and retrieved with *loadModel()* functions of the module, which are not shown in the listing). The new data, on which classification should be performed, is retrieved from database, where data is inserted by system user filling a suitable *New patient* form through the application interface (see Fig. 10.1). Predicted category is returned by *predict()* function and presented to the user, as *Prediction report*.

Listing 10.1 Prototype classification module for RECTIN system.

```
1    package classification;
2
3    import weka.classifiers.bayes.NaiveBayes;
4    import weka.classifiers.meta.FilteredClassifier;
5    import weka.attributeSelection.AttributeSelection;
6    import weka.attributeSelection.ChiSquaredAttributeEval;
7    import weka.attributeSelection.Ranker;
8    import weka.core.converters.ConverterUtils.DataSource;
9    import weka.experiment.InstanceQuery;
10   import weka.filters.Filter;
11   import weka.filters.unsupervised.attribute.Remove;
12   import weka.core.Instances;
13   /**
14    * Module implementing classification model learning
15    * and prediction on new data.
16    */
17   public class Classification{
18       /*
19        * Main class calls learn and predict method.
20        */
21       public static void main(String[] args) throws Exception{
22           Filter filter = learn();
23           System.out.println(predict(filter));
24       }
25       /**
26        * Learns prediction model based on data in csv file.
27        * Saves model to file.
28        * @return Filter that selects attributes
29        */
30       public static Filter learn() throws Exception{
31
32           DataSource source =
33           new DataSource("classification/data/pred_vis0.csv");
34           Instances data = source.getDataSet();
35
36           if (data.classIndex() == -1)
```

```
37                     data.setClassIndex(data.numAttributes() - 1);
38
39          FilteredClassifier classifier = new FilteredClassifier();
40          //set attribute filter to use on new data
41          AttributeSelection filter = new AttributeSelection();
42          // package weka.filters.supervised.attribute!
43          ChiSquaredAttributeEval eval =
44          new ChiSquaredAttributeEval();
45          Ranker search = new Ranker();
46          search.setNumToSelect(80);
47          filter.setEvaluator(eval);
48          filter.setSearch(search);
49          filter.SelectAttributes(data);
50
51          int[] retArr = filter.selectedAttributes();
52
53          //set up the filter for removing attributes
54          Filter remove = new Remove();
55          ((Remove) remove).setAttributeIndicesArray(retArr);
56          ((Remove) remove).setInvertSelection(true);
57          //retain the selected,remove all others
58          remove.setInputFormat(data);
59          Instances newData = Filter.useFilter(data, remove);
60
61          NaiveBayes nB = new NaiveBayes();
62          classifier.setClassifier(nB);
63          classifier.buildClassifier(newData);
64
65          //dump meta-classifier
66          saveModel(classifier, "NB80", "classification/models/");
67          /*
68           * Evaluation
69          Evaluation evaluation = new Evaluation(data);
70          evaluation.crossValidateModel(nB, newData, 10, new Random(1));
71          System.out.println(evaluation.toSummaryString());
72           */
73          return remove;
74          }
75      /**
76       * Performs prediction based on saved model.
77       * Returns predicted category.
78       * @param Filter selector for attributes on new data
79       * @return predicted category
80       */
81      public static double predict(Filter selector) throws Exception{
82          /*
83           * Load prediction model
84           */
85          FilteredClassifier classifier =
86          loadModel("classification/models/","NB80");
87          /*
88           * Perform prediction on new data
89           */
```

```
90          InstanceQuery queryNewData = new InstanceQuery();
91          queryNewData.setQuery
92          ("select top 2 * from Tinnitus.dbo.finalPred6");
93          Instances unlabeled = queryNewData.retrieveInstances();
94          Instances newData = Filter.useFilter(unlabeled, selector);
95          // set class attribute
96          newData.setClassIndex(newData.numAttributes() - 1);
97          newData.instance(0).setClassMissing();
98
99          double label =
100         classifier.classifyInstance(newData.instance(0));
101         System.out.print
102         ("predicted category: "+
103          newData.classAttribute().value((int) label));
104
105         return (label);
106     }
107 }
```

10.4 Rule Engine

Rule Engine module prototype, as a component of application architecture depicted in Fig. 10.1, is implemented in the Java Platform with the use of Jess library (the Rule Engine for the Java Platform) [FH+08].

To use the library for diagnostic and treatment recommendation purposes, decision and action rules obtained in experiments have to be specified in the form of rules using either XML format or the Jess rule language. Examples of diagnostic and treatment rules specified in the former format are presented in Listings 10.2 and 10.3. Whenever new rules are extracted, they can be easily added to the system logic. This is done by writing explicit "diagnosis" and "treatment" libraries (*diagnosis.clp* and *treatment.clp* files), which then can be invoked from a Web application or from Java code.

Listing 10.2 Sample diagnostic rules declaration (diagnosis.clp) for Rule Engine Module in RECTIN System.

```
1   ;; First define templates for the model classes so we can use them
2   ;; in our diagnostic rules. This doesn't create any model objects--
3   ;; it just tells Jess to examine the classes and set up templates
4   ;; using their properties
5
6   (import ruleEngine.diagnosis.model.*)
7   (deftemplate Visit        (declare (from-class Visit)))
8   (deftemplate VisitItem    (declare (from-class VisitItem)))
9   (deftemplate Diagnosis (declare (from-class DiagnosisItem)))
10  (deftemplate Patient      (declare (from-class Patient)))
11
12  ;; Now define the diagnosis rules themselves. Each rule matches a set
13  ;; of conditions and then creates an Diagnosis object to represent a
```

```
14   ;; diagnosis recommendation to a patient. The rules assume that
15   ;; there will be just one Visit, its VisitsItems, and its Patient in
16   ;; working memory, along with all the Diagnosis objects.
17
18
19   (defrule C0-LSD_LL4_LR8_RSD
20      'Diagnose with Category 0 if audiological evaluation of L SD >=100,
21      LL4 >=999, LR8 >=999,R SD >=100'
22      (VisitItem {LSD >= 100})
23      (VisitItem {LL4 >= 999})
24      (VisitItem {LR8 >= 999})
25      (VisitItem {R SD >=100})
26      =>
27      (add (new Diagnosis'Category 0, 50% conf.' 0 50)))
28
29   (defrule C1-R3-TAn
30      'Diagnose with Category 1 if audiological evaluation of 20 > R3 >=15,
31      tinnitus annoyance as indicated in Interview Questionnaire >=8.'
32      (VisitItem {R3 >= 15 && R3 < 20})
33      (VisitItem {T_An >=8})
34      =>
35      (add (new Diagnosis'Category 1, 94% conf.' 1 94)))
36
37   (defrule C2-HLpr
38      'Diagnose with Category 2 if hearing loss problem,
39      as indicated in Interview Questionnaire, >=5.'
40      (VisitItem {HL_pr >= 5})
41      =>
42      (add (new Diagnosis'Category 2, 54% conf.' 2 54)))
43
44   (defrule C3-LL3-Hpr_HSv
45      'Diagnose with Category 3 if audiological evaluation of 91>LL3 >=85,
46      hyperacusis problem as indicated in Interview Questionnaire >=7,
47      hyperacusis severity as indicated in Interview Questionnaire >=7.5'
48      (VisitItem {LL3 >= 85 && LL3 < 91})
49      (VisitItem {H_pr >=7})
50      (VisitItem {H_Sv >=7.5})
51      =>
52      (add (new Diagnosis'Category 3, 100% conf.' 3 100)))
53
54   (defrule C4-LSD_L4_LL3
55      'Diagnose with Category 4 if audiological evaluation of L SD >=100,
56      L4 <10, LL3 <75'
57      (VisitItem {LSD >= 100})
58      (VisitItem {L4 < 10})
59      (VisitItem {LL3 <75})
60      =>
61      (add (new Diagnosis'Category 4, 67% conf.' 4 67)))
```

Listing 10.3 Sample treatment rules declaration (treatment.clp) for Rule Engine Module in RECTIN System.

```
1   (import ruleEngine.treatment.model.*)
2   (deftemplate Visit      (declare (from-class Visit)))
```

```
3    (deftemplate VisitItem    (declare (from-class VisitItem)))
4    (deftemplate Treatment (declare (from-class TreatmentItem)))
5    (deftemplate Patient      (declare (from-class Patient)))
6
7    (defrule Instr_GHI_Freq_LE
8       'Change Freq LE setting of GHI instrument from 3000-3150
9       to higher than 3775,
10      to increase improvement by 32\% points'
11      (VisitItem {Instr GHI})
12      (VisitItem {Freq_LE >= 3000 && Freq_LE < 3150))
13      =>
14      (add (new Treatment'GHI Freq LE -> >=3775, impr. 32 pp.' 32)))
15
16   (defrule CC0_CC1
17      'Change treatment protocol in patient diagnosed with C0
18      from CC0 to CC1
19      to increase improvement by 33\% points'
20      (VisitItem {Cat 0})
21      (VisitItem {CC 0})
22      =>
23      (add (new Treatment'CC -> 1, impr. 33 pp.' 33)))
24
25   (defrule Age_G_Cat_Tside_MendNr
26      'For a male patient diagnosed with C1
27      whose tinntius began at age 50-55 as outcome of medicaments,
28      decrease number of medications patient takes from 5 to at most 2
29      to increase improvement by 55\% points'
30      (VisitItem {AgeBeg>=50 && AgeBeg<55})
31      (VisitItem {G m})
32      (VisitItem {Cat 1})
33      (VisitItem {T_side 1})
34      (VisitItem {Med_nr >= 5})
35      =>
36      (add (new Treatment'MedNr -> 2, impr. 55 pp.' 55)))
37
38   (defrule NTI_G_Instr
39      'For a male patient whose tinnitus onset associated with noise
40      change instrumentation from GH soft to GH hard
41      to increase improvement by 33\% points'
42      (VisitItem {NTI 1})
43      (VisitItem {G m})
44      (VisitItem {Instr GHS})
45      =>
46      (add (new Treatment'Instr -> GHH, impr.33pp.' 33)))
47
48   (defrule G_Tside_Ulcers
49      'For male patients with ulcers living in Georgia state
50      whose tinnitus onset associated with medications
51      decrease number of medication, recommend moving to Illinois
52      to increase improvement by 73\% points'
53      (VisitItem {T_side 1})
54      (VisitItem {G m})
55      (VisitItem {Ulcers 1})
```

```
56      (VisitItem {Med_nr >= 5})
57      =>
58      (add (new Treatment'MedNr -> 2, State -> IL, impr. 73 pp.' 73)))
```

10.4.1 Rete Algorithm for Rule Execution

The Rete algorithm described in [For82] became the basis for a whole generation of fast rule engines. The algorithm is implemented by building a network of nodes, each of which represents one or more tests found on a rule LHS. Facts that are being added to or removed from the working memory are processed by this network of nodes. At the bottom of the network there are nodes representing individual rules. When a set of facts filters all the way down to the bottom of the network, it has passed all the tests on the LHS of a particular rule and this set becomes an *activation*. The associated rule may have its RHS executed (*fired*) if the activation is not invalidated first by the removal of one or more facts from its activation set.

Example rules, as depicted below

```
(defrule example-2        (defrule example-3
    (x)                       (x)
    (y)                       (y)
    (z)                       => )
    => )
```

are compiled into the network as depicted in Fig. 10.3.

The nodes marked x?, etc., test if a fact contains the given data, while the nodes marked + remember all facts and fire whenever they have received data from both their left and right inputs. To run the network, Jess presents new facts to each node at the top of the network as they are added to the working memory. Each node takes input from the top and sends its output downwards. A single input node generally

Fig. 10.3 Illustration of RETE algorithm used in RECTIN Rule Engine [FH+08]

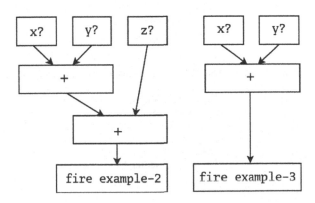

receives a fact from above, applies a test to it, and, if the test passes, sends the fact downward to the next node. If the test fails, the one-input nodes simply do nothing. The two-input nodes have to integrate facts from their left and right inputs. The two input nodes must remember all facts that are presented to them, and attempt to group facts arriving on their left inputs with facts arriving on their right inputs to make up complete activation sets. A two-input node therefore has a *left memory* and a *right memory* [FH+08].

Rule execution procedure for *Rule Engine* module in RECTIN is implemented with the Rete Algorithm (see Listing 10.4). The Java code presented in the listing creates an instance of the Jess rule engine, loads in the visit data, then loads in the rules. This one instance of Jess can be reused to process each patient/visit. The engine is supposed to look at each visit data (with audiological evaluation, form responses, etc.), together with a patient's data (demographics, tinnitus induction, visit history), and apply diagnosis and different treatment actions to the recommendation given to a physician. The diagnosis engine's decision method takes a visit identifier and returns an *Iterator* over all applicable decisions (diagnoses). Rules are matched against simple Java model objects (*Patient, Visit, VisitItem, Diagnosis, Treatment*). With the use of Jess's predefined *Filter* implementations, only one *Diagnosis* object is selected from working memory.

Listing 10.4 Prototype rule engine for RECTIN system.

```
1    package ruleEngine.diagnosis;
2
3    import ruleEngine.diagnosis.model.Diagnosis;
4    import ruleEngine.diagnosis.model.Visit;
5    import jess.*;
6
7    import java.util.Iterator;
8
9    public class DiagnosisEngine {
10       private Rete engine;
11       private WorkingMemoryMarker marker;
12       private Database database;
13
14       public DiagnosisEngine(Database aDatabase) throws JessException {
15           // Create a Jess rule engine
16           engine = new Rete();
17           engine.reset();
18
19           // Load the diagnosis rules
20           engine.batch("diagnosis.clp");
21
22           // Load the Diagnosis data into working memory
23           database = aDatabase;
24           engine.addAll(database.getDiagnosisItems());
25
26           // Mark end of diagnosis data for later
27           marker = engine.mark();
28       }
29
```

```
30      private void loadVisitData(int visitId) throws JessException {
31          // Retrieve the visit from the database
32          Visit visit = database.getVisit(visitId);
33
34          if (visit != null) {
35              // Add the visitand its contents to working memory
36              engine.add(visit);
37              engine.add(visit.getPatient());
38              engine.addAll(visit.getItems());
39          }
40      }
41
42      public Iterator run(int visitId) throws JessException {
43          // Remove any previous visit data, leaving only diagnosis data
44          engine.resetToMark(marker);
45
46          // Load data for this visit
47          loadVisitData(visitId);
48
49          // Fire the rules that apply to this visit
50          engine.run();
51
52          // Return the list of diagnoses created by the rules
53          return engine.getObjects(new Filter.ByClass(Diagnosis.class));
54      }
55  }
```

10.5   Conclusion

Prototype implementation described in this chapter serves as a basis for full RECTIN implementation. It illustrates basic mechanisms on which system functionalities should be based. It must be taken into account that programming the whole application and database part, as well as defining knowledge base consisting of relevant rules is a project of few months work. It should involve cooperation with potential users and organization where the system should be deployed so that to tailor it to their specific needs. The proposed system is scalable and flexible. Knowledge base and prediction models are assumed to relearn with the new medical knowledge entered into the RECTIN database. New rules and better prediction models should be developed with new available data.

Chapter 11
Final Conclusions and Future Work

Abstract This book presented a process of analysis, design and prototype implementation of RECTIN recommender system, as a solution to the problem of supporting tinnitus treatment based on Tinnitus Retraining Therapy in a medical facility. Proposed approach in supporting physicians' diagnosis and treatment decisions addresses scarcity of expert knowledge, time restrictions in today's medical practice and the need for more efficient evaluation of different treatment methods. Such system can provide accurate support at any time, with full consideration of individual patient profiles, including: demographics, medical history, and tinnitus background.

11.1 Objective Verification

This book presented a process of analysis, design and prototype implementation of RECTIN recommender system, as a solution to the problem of supporting tinnitus treatment based on Tinnitus Retraining Therapy in a medical facility. Proposed approach in supporting physicians' diagnosis and treatment decisions addresses scarcity of expert knowledge, time restrictions in today's medical practice and the need for more efficient evaluation of different treatment methods. Such system can provide accurate support at any time, with full consideration of individual patient profiles, including: demographics, medical history, and tinnitus background.

The work within this book verifies a hypothesis about possibility to apply theory of traditional machine learning techniques, such as classification and association rules, as well as novel data mining methods, including action rules and meta actions, to a practical decision problem in the area of medicine. In particular, authors investigated knowledge discovery approach in order to build rule-based recommender system for tinnitus treatment and diagnosis.

© Springer International Publishing AG 2017
K.A. Tarnowska et al., *Decision Support System for Diagnosis and Treatment of Hearing Disorders*, Studies in Computational Intelligence 685,
DOI 10.1007/978-3-319-51463-5_11

The work started with analysis of medical and social aspects of tinnitus problem, focusing on the successful treatment method—Tinnitus Retraining Therapy developed by doctor Jastreboff from Emory University School of Medicine in Atlanta. The effectiveness of the method and availability of the dataset of patients treated with it, provided major motivation for taking up the project for developing decision support system with knowledge base in this area.

After introduction to the problem area and preliminary analysis of available dataset, an overview of available methods for recommender system's development was discussed. Different approaches have been described and compared. Major application areas of RS were also presented, in the context of their technical deployments and practical usage. This helped in initial choice of a method and design of RS for a given problem area. Chosen methodology of knowledge-based recommendation was expanded with elaboration on theoretical background of knowledge discovery methods, including concepts, such as: Information System, Decision Tables, Reducts, Action Rules and Meta Actions, with their possible application to the medical dataset. Techniques of dealing with temporal visit data were also described, including advanced clustering techniques.

Based on the given problem area, researched solutions for recommendation systems and detailed theoretical algorithms for knowledge discovery, an architecture of Recommender System for Tinnitus Treatment and Diagnosis (RECTIN) was proposed and described. Each component of the system was presented in deployment details, but the main focus was knowledge engineering phase in the system development. This step included a series of data preprocessing steps, new feature development and empirical tests on data mining with the chosen methodologies and tools. Tests on knowledge discovery were divided into: classifier testing, decision rule extraction and action rules/meta action generation. New flexible temporal features were developed to describe the sparse visiting records of patients for the purpose of classification model construction and action rule discovery. Interesting and potentially novel action rules about the relationship among treatment factors and symptoms were revealed. The experiment's outcomes provided basis for prototype RECTIN system implementation with further possibilities of its extension.

11.2 Further Work

Further work in this project includes: full implementation of RECTIN system and validity tests on unseen cases of new patients willing to treat their tinnitus with TRT methodology, which is definitely needed, from medical point of view. The system would apply rules discovered in this study to input data on the patient during each visit. The recommendation for the patient treatment would be based on the placement of the current patient state to the action rules suggesting treatment patterns to the physician. Verification and testing of a built prototype performed with experiments on new cases of patients data would make a base for further analysis and description of research results, as well as, assessing the quality of the solution. Hybrid techniques of recommender system technology can be also used to enhance the proposed approach, including collaborative filtering and content-based recommendation.

Experiments on data mining should be continued so that to improve the knowledge domain for the recommender system. It is expected that as database grows and more examples are collected, the confidence and support of the decision/action rules will increase. Experiments on the new extended database, which could help in discovering relations between emotional changes in patients and their tinnitus symptoms, would be of particular interest. Further work on text mining can be performed, as well as clustering techniques, which introduce homogeneity to the dataset based on time between visits and number of visits.

Finally, approach presented in this work should not be limited to the decision problems related with tinnitus diagnosis and treatment, and health care area, in general. As presented in Chap. 3, recommender systems are currently implemented in practically every aspect of people's life, worldwide, on the grounds of the competitive advantage resulting from their implementation and usage. Action rules present a promising approach for building recommender systems. Since its introduction in 2000, they have been successfully applied in many domain areas. Strategic importance of recommender systems based on action rules results from their potential to increase efficiency and effectiveness of decision-making processes. Action rules help to analyze data to improve understanding of it and seek specific actions (recommendations) to enhance the decision-making process. In the long-term, improvement of decision-making processes leads to growth of the whole organization and its profitability. On the other hand, organizations that do not implement modern technologies based on intelligent systems will face difficulties in further growth or even survival in the knowledge-based economy. Technology of recommender systems is developing very quickly as a modern method of machine reasoning and learning, infiltrating from academics and research to practical applications. Recommendation approach based on actions presents a new way in machine learning, which solves problems that traditional methods cannot handle.

Appendix A
Tinnitus Initial Interview Form

TINNITUS / HYPERACUSIS
INITIAL INTERVIEW FORM

Clinic # :
Name :
DOB :
SSN :
Insurance :
Date :

T&HC#:

tel:
e-mail:

TINNITUS

RE / LE / Both / Head = > Intermittent / Constant
Onset: Gradual / Sudden When
Fluctuations in volume Y / N
Description of T sound(s)

"Bad days" Y / N Frequency

Activities prevented or affected:
○Concentration ○Sleep ○QRA ○Work
○Restaurants ○Sports ○Social ○Other

Effect of sound: None / Louder / Softer
How long: min / hours / days

Ear overprotection Y / N % of time
in quiet Y / N

% of time when: Aware Annoyed
Severity: 0 1 2 3 4 5 6 7 8 9 10
Annoyance: 0 1 2 3 4 5 6 7 8 9 10
Effect on Life: 0 1 2 3 4 5 6 7 8 9 10

Any other T specific treatments

Why is T a problem

Comments:

SOUND TOLERANCE

Oversensitivity: Y / N Physical discomfort? Y / N
Description of troublesome sounds

"Bad days" Y / N Frequency

Activities prevented or affected:
○Concerts ○Shopping ○Movies ○Work
○Restaurants ○Driving ○Sports ○Church
○Housekeeping ○Childcare ○Social ○Other

Effect of sound: None / Stronger / Weaker
How long: min / hours / days

Ear overprotection Y / N % of time
in quiet Y / N

Severity: 0 1 2 3 4 5 6 7 8 9 10
Annoyance: 0 1 2 3 4 5 6 7 8 9 10
Effect on Life: 0 1 2 3 4 5 6 7 8 9 10

Any other ST specific treatments

Why is ST a problem

Comments:

HL

Hearing problem Y / N
Hearing Aid(s) Y / N type:
Ever recommended Y / N

Category:
Recommendation:

Ranking problems: Tinnitus: 0 1 2 3 4 5
Sound tolerance: 0 1 2 3 4 5
Hearing: 0 1 2 3 4 5

Ptn decision:
Next visit:

T - tinnitus ST - sound tolerance (hyperacusis + phonophobia)
Is you T preventing or affecting any activities in your life.
QRA - quiet recreational activities: Is your T interfering with QRA such as reading or meditating.
% of time when: Aware - What % of time were you aware of your T over last month?
Annoyed - What % of the time over last months T bothered you?
Severity - How strong or loud is your T on average over last month? 0 - no T, 10 - as strong as you can imagine.
Annoyance - How much was T annoying you on average over last month 0 - not at all; 10 - as much as you can imagine.
Effect on life - How much was T affecting your life on average over last month. 0 - no effect; 10 - as much as you can imagine.
Any other T specific treatments - Are you using any other treatments for your T.
Sound tolerance - Is your tolerance to louder sounds the same as people around you?
Hearing - Do you think you have a hearing problem?
Ranking - rank importance of your problems with 0 - no problem, 5 - as large as you can imagine

MM & PJ Jastreboff, 1999

© Springer International Publishing AG 2017
K.A. Tarnowska et al., *Decision Support System for Diagnosis and Treatment of Hearing Disorders*, Studies in Computational Intelligence 685, DOI 10.1007/978-3-319-51463-5

Appendix B
Tinnitus Follow-up Interview Form

FU

TINNITUS / HYPERACUSIS
FOLLOW-UP INTERVIEW FORM

CATEGORY:
Date of init. couns.
T&HC#:   Date of instr. fitt.
           SG:
tel: HA:
           FUQ #:
           Month #:

Clinic #   :
Name   :
DOB   :
SSN   :
Insurance :
Date   :

TINNITUS

Activities prevented or affected: Changes: Y / N
◯◯Concentration ◯◯Sleep   ◯◯QRA ◯◯Work
◯◯Restaurants   ◯◯Sports   ◯◯Social ◯◯Other

% of time when: Aware   (1st) Annoyed   (1st)
Has it changed
Severity: 0 1 2 3 4 5 6 7 8 9 10
Annoyance: 0 1 2 3 4 5 6 7 8 9 10
Effect on Life: 0 1 2 3 4 5 6 7 8 9 10

Comments:

"Bad days" Y / N   Frequency
Are they: as frequent Y /N   as bad Y / N

Effect of sound: None / Louder / Softer
         How long: min / hours / days

Ear overprotection Y / N   % of time
              in quiet Y / N
Any other T specific treatments

SOUND TOLERANCE
H
L

Description of troublesome sounds

Activities prevented or affected: Changes: Y / N
◯◯Concerts   ◯◯Shopping ◯◯Movies ◯◯Work
◯◯Restaurants   ◯◯Driving   ◯◯Sports ◯◯Church
◯◯Housekeeping ◯◯Childcare ◯◯Social ◯◯Other

Severity: 0 1 2 3 4 5 6 7 8 9 10
Annoyance: 0 1 2 3 4 5 6 7 8 9 10
Effect on Life: 0 1 2 3 4 5 6 7 8 9 10

Comments:

"Bad days" Y / N   Frequency
Are they: as frequent Y /N   as bad Y / N

Effect of sound: None / Stronger/ Weaker
         How long: min / hours / days

Ear overprotection Y / N   % of time
              in quiet Y / N
Any other ST specific treatments

Hearing problem

Recommendation:

The problem in general: Same / Better / Worse
Ranking problems: Tinnitus: 0 1 2 3 4 5
               Sound tolerance: 0 1 2 3 4 5
                    Hearing: 0 1 2 3 4 5

Next visit:

How would you feel if you had to give back your instruments
Are you glad you started this program? Y / N / NS

Main problems discussed:

T - tinnitus   ST - sound tolerance (hyperacusis + phonophobia)
Is you T preventing or affecting any activities in your life.
QRA - quiet recreational activities: Is your T interfering with QRA such as reading or meditating.
today
% of time when: Aware - What % of time were you aware of your T over last month?
          Annoyed - What % of the time over last months T bothered you?
Severity - How strong or loud is your T on average over last month? 0 - no T, 10 - as strong as you can imagine.
Annoyance - How much was T annoying you on average over last month 0 - not at all; 10 - as much as you can imagine.
Effect on life - How much was T affecting your life on average over last month. 0 - no effect; 10 - as much as you can imagine.
Any other T specific treatments - Are you using any other treatments for your T.
Sound tolerance - Is your tolerance to louder sounds the same as people around you?
Hearing - Do you think you have a hearing problem?
Ranking - rank importance of your problems with 0 - no problem, 5 - as large as you can imagine
1999

●◯ - an activity affected at first visit
◯● - an activity affected as for

MM & PJ Jastreboff,

MM & PJ Jastreboff,

© Springer International Publishing AG 2017
K.A. Tarnowska et al., *Decision Support System for Diagnosis and Treatment of Hearing Disorders*, Studies in Computational Intelligence 685,
DOI 10.1007/978-3-319-51463-5

Appendix C
Tinnitus Handicap Inventory

Tinnitus Handicap Inventory (THI)

This form is for informational purposes only and should not take the place of consultation and evaluation by a healthcare professional.

Your Name: _____ Date: _____

Instructions: The purpose of this questionnaire is to identify, quantify, and evaluate the difficulties that you may be experiencing because of tinnitus. Please do not skip any questions. When you have answer all the questions, add up your total score, based on the values for each response.

1. Because of your tinnitus, is it difficult for you to concentrate?	○ Yes (4) ○ Sometimes (2) ○ No (0)	
2. Does the loudness of your tinnitus make it difficult for you to hear people?	○ Yes (4) ○ Sometimes (2) ○ No (0)	
3. Does your tinnitus make you angry?	○ Yes (4) ○ Sometimes (2) ○ No (0)	
4. Does your tinnitus make you feel confused?	○ Yes (4) ○ Sometimes (2) ○ No (0)	
5. Because of your tinnitus, do you feel desperate?	○ Yes (4) ○ Sometimes (2) ○ No (0)	
6. Do you complain a great deal about your tinnitus?	○ Yes (4) ○ Sometimes (2) ○ No (0)	
7. Because of your tinnitus, do you have trouble falling to sleep at night?	○ Yes (4) ○ Sometimes (2) ○ No (0)	
8. Do you feel as though you cannot escape your tinnitus?	○ Yes (4) ○ Sometimes (2) ○ No (0)	
9. Does your tinnitus interfere with your ability to enjoy your social activities (such as going out to dinner, to the movies)?	○ Yes (4) ○ Sometimes (2) ○ No (0)	
10. Because of your tinnitus, do you feel frustrated?	○ Yes (4) ○ Sometimes (2) ○ No (0)	
11. Because of your tinnitus, do you feel that you have a terrible disease?	○ Yes (4) ○ Sometimes (2) ○ No (0)	
12. Does your tinnitus make it difficult for you to enjoy life?	○ Yes (4) ○ Sometimes (2) ○ No (0)	
13. Does your tinnitus interfere with your job or household responsibilities?	○ Yes (4) ○ Sometimes (2) ○ No (0)	
14. Because of your tinnitus, do you find that you are often irritable?	○ Yes (4) ○ Sometimes (2) ○ No (0)	
15. Because of your tinnitus, is it difficult for you to read?	○ Yes (4) ○ Sometimes (2) ○ No (0)	
16. Does your tinnitus make you upset?	○ Yes (4) ○ Sometimes (2) ○ No (0)	
17. Do you feel that your tinnitus problem has placed stress on your relationships with members of your family and friends?	○ Yes (4) ○ Sometimes (2) ○ No (0)	
18. Do you find it difficult to focus your attention away from your tinnitus and on other things?	○ Yes (4) ○ Sometimes (2) ○ No (0)	
19. Do you feel that you have no control over your tinnitus?	○ Yes (4) ○ Sometimes (2) ○ No (0)	
20. Because of your tinnitus, do you often feel tired?	○ Yes (4) ○ Sometimes (2) ○ No (0)	
21. Because of your tinnitus, do you feel depressed?	○ Yes (4) ○ Sometimes (2) ○ No (0)	
22. Does your tinnitus make you feel anxious?	○ Yes (4) ○ Sometimes (2) ○ No (0)	
23. Do you feel that you can no longer cope with your tinnitus?	○ Yes (4) ○ Sometimes (2) ○ No (0)	
24. Does your tinnitus get worse when you are under stress?	○ Yes (4) ○ Sometimes (2) ○ No (0)	
25. Does your tinnitus make you feel insecure?	○ Yes (4) ○ Sometimes (2) ○ No (0)	

The sum of all responses is your THI Score >>> | 0 |

0-16: Slight or no handicap (Grade 1)
18-36: Mild handicap (Grade 2)
38-56: Moderate handicap (Grade 3)
58-76: Severe handicap (Grade 4)
78-100: Catastrophic handicap (Grade 5)

Newman CW, Jacobson GP, Spitzer JB. (1996) "Development of the Tinnitus Handicap Inventory."
Archives of Otolaryngology - Head and Neck Surgery. 122(2):143-8.
McCombe, A., Baguley, D., Coles, R., McKenna, L., McKinney, C. & Windle-Taylor, P. (2001). "Guidelines for the Grading of Tinnitus Severity: the Results of a Working Group Commissioned by the British Association of Otolaryngologists, Head and Neck Surgeons." Clinical Otolaryngology 26, 388-393.

© Springer International Publishing AG 2017
K.A. Tarnowska et al., *Decision Support System for Diagnosis and Treatment of Hearing Disorders*, Studies in Computational Intelligence 685, DOI 10.1007/978-3-319-51463-5

References

[AT05]   Adomavicius, Gediminas; Tuzhilin, Alexander: Toward the next generation of recommender systems: A survey of the state-of-the-art and possible extensions. In: *Knowledge and Data Engineering, IEEE Transactions on* 17 (2005), Nr. 6, pp. 734–749

[BFH+14]   Bouckaert, Remco R.; Frank, Eibe; Hall, Mark ; Kirkby, Richard; Reutemann, Peter; Seewald, Alex; Scuse, David. *WEKA Manual for Version 3-6-12*. 2014

[FH+08]   Friedman-Hill, Ernest [u. a.]. *Jess, the rule engine for the java platform*. 2008

[FISZ07]   Felfernig, Alexander; Isak, Klaus; Szabo, Kalman; Zachar, Peter: The VITA financial services sales support environment. In: *PROCEEDINGS OF THE NATIONAL CONFERENCE ON ARTIFICIAL INTELLIGENCE* Bd. 22 Menlo Park, CA; Cambridge, MA; London; AAAI Press; MIT Press; 1999, 2007, pp. 1692

[For82]   Forgy, Charles L.: Rete: A fast algorithm for the many pattern/many object pattern match problem. In: *Artificial intelligence* 19 (1982), Nr. 1, pp. 17–37

[HS10]   Hassan, Shahzaib; Syed, Zeeshan: From netflix to heart attacks: collaborative filtering in medical datasets. In: *Proceedings of the 1st ACM International Health Informatics Symposium* ACM, 2010, pp. 128–134

[IR08]   Im, Seunghyun; Ras, Zbigniew W.: Action rule extraction from a decision table: ARED. In: *Foundations of Intelligent Systems*. Springer, 2008, pp. 160–168

[IRT11]   Im, Seunghyun; Ras, Zbigniew; Tsay, Li-Shiang: Action reducts. In: *Foundations of Intelligent Systems*. Springer, 2011, pp. 62–69

[JH04]   Jastreboff, Pawel J.; Hazell, Jonathan W.: *Tinnitus retraining therapy: implementing the neurophysiological model*. Cambridge University Press, 2004

[JJ00]   Jastreboff, Pawel J.; Jastreboff, Margaret M.: Tinnitus retraining therapy (TRT) as a method for treatment of tinnitus and hyperacusis patients. In: *JOURNAL-AMERICAN ACADEMY OF AUDIOLOGY* 11 (2000), Nr. 3, pp. 162–177

[JJ06]   Jastreboff, Pawel J.; Jastreboff, Margaret M.: Tinnitus retraining therapy: a different view on tinnitus. In: *Orl* 68 (2006), Nr. 1, pp. 23–30

[JZFF10]   Jannach, Dietmar; Zanker, Markus; Felfernig, Alexander; Friedrich, Gerhard: *Recommender systems: an introduction*. Cambridge University Press, 2010

[KDJR14]   Kuang, Jieyan; Daniel, Albert; Johnston, Jill; Ras, Zbigniew W.: Hierarchically Structured Recommender System for Improving NPS of a Company. In: *Rough Sets and Current Trends in Computing* Springer, 2014, pp. 347–357

[KP08]   Khosrow-Pour, Mehdi: *Encyclopedia of information science and technology*. Bd. 1. IGI Global, 2008

© Springer International Publishing AG 2017

K.A. Tarnowska et al., *Decision Support System for Diagnosis and Treatment of Hearing Disorders*, Studies in Computational Intelligence 685, DOI 10.1007/978-3-319-51463-5

[KRRS11]   Kantor, Paul B.; Rokach, Lior; Ricci, Francesco; Shapira, Bracha: *Recommender systems handbook*. Springer, 2011

[MLDK10]   Møller, Aage R.; Langguth, Berthold; DeRidder, Dirk; Kleinjung, Tobias: *Textbook of tinnitus*. Springer Science & Business Media, 2010

[Nek]   Nekvapil, Viktor: USING THE AC4FT-MINER PROCEDURE IN THE MEDICAL DOMAIN.

[Paw85]   Pawlak, Zdzislaw: Rough sets and decision tables. In: *Computation Theory*. Springer, 1985, pp. 187–196

[PM81]   Pawlak, Zdzislaw ; Marek, W: Rough sets and information systems. In: *ICS. PAS. Reports (441)* (1981), pp. 481–485

[Ras15]   Ras, Zbigniew W.: *Action Rules and Meta Actions*. http://www.cs.uncc.edu/~ras/ ActionRules.ppt. 2015. – [Online; accessed 20-May-2015]

[RD09]   Ras, Zbigniew W.; Dardzinska, Agnieszka: Action rules discovery based on tree classifiers and meta-actions. In: *Foundations of Intelligent Systems*. Springer, 2009, pp. 66–75

[RDTW08]   Ras, Zbigniew W.; Dardzinska, Agnieszka; Tsay, Li-Shiang; Wasyluk, Hanna: Association action rules. In: *Data Mining Workshops, 2008. ICDMW'08. IEEE International Conference on* IEEE, 2008, pp. 283–290

[RW00]   Ras, Zbigniew W.; Wieczorkowska, Alicja: Action-rules: How to increase profit of a company. In: *Principles of Data Mining and Knowledge Discovery*. Springer, 2000, pp. 587–592

[Sim14]   Simunek, Milan: LISp-Miner Control Language description of scripting language implementation. In: *Journal of Systems Integration* 5 (2014), Nr. 2, pp. 28–44

[SK13]   Sodsee, Sunantha; Komkhao, Maytiyanin: Evidence-based Medical Recommender Systems: A Review. In: *International Journal of Information Processing & Management* 4 (2013), Nr. 6

[Szl15]   Szlufik, K. Ciecierski R. Rola T. Mandat P. Nauman Z. Ras A. Przybyszewski A. Friedman D. K.: DBS decision support system based on analysis of microelectrode recorded signals as an useful tool in detection of the most beneficial electrode localization during DBS implantation. In: *Brain Stimulation* 8 (2015), Nr. 2, pp. 396–397

[Tho11]   Thompson, Pamela Liberty M.: *Mining for knowledge to build decision support system for diagnosis and treatment of tinnitus*, University of North Carolina at Charlotte, Diss., 2011

[TKHR13]   Touati, Hakim; Kuang, Jieyan; Hajja, Ayman; Ras, Zbigniew W.: Personalized action rules for side effects object grouping. (2013)

[TRSW14]   Touati, Hakim; Ras, Zbigniew W.; Studnicki, James; Wieczorkowska, Alicja: Mining Surgical Meta-actions Effects with Variable Diagnoses' Number. In: *Foundations of Intelligent Systems*. Springer, 2014, pp. 254–263

[Wan14]   Wang, John: *Encyclopedia of Business Analytics and Optimization*. IGI Global, 2014

[Web15]   Webb, Jonathan: *Tinnitus mapped inside human brain*. http://www.bbc.com/news/ science-environment-32414876. 2015. – [Online; accessed 15-May-2015]

[WP14]   Wiesner, Martin; Pfeifer, Daniel: Health recommender systems: Concepts, requirements, technical basics and challenges. In: *International journal of environmental research and public health* 11 (2014), Nr. 3, pp. 2580–2607

[ZRJT10]   Zhang, Xin; Ras, Zbigniew W.; Jastreboff, Pawel J.; Thompson, Pamela L.: From tinnitus data to action rules and tinnitus treatment. In: *Granular Computing (GrC), 2010 IEEE International Conference on* IEEE, 2010, pp. 620–625

Printed in the United States
By Bookmasters